Parenting a Child

on the

Spectrum

2

Where Are They Now?

Compiled by Deborah Fay

Table of Contents

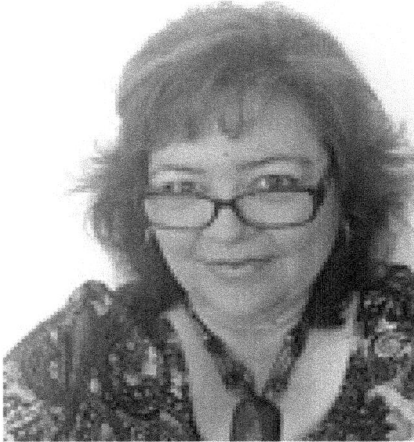

Introduction
by Deborah Fay

Four years ago, I very proudly launched *Parenting a Child on the Spectrum – Inspiring accounts of the ups and downs that go with parenting a child with Autism* and I could not have been happier with the physical outcome of a vision I'd held for almost 15 years.

What an experience! With contributions from authors all over Australia we had a great time writing, compiling, editing, publishing and then launching the book. Many of the authors were able to join us at the official launch which was massive.

The Captain Cook Bridge in the heart of Brisbane city was 'lit up blue' for Autism and for the launch of our book. We then had radio interviews all around Southeast Queensland, including with the ABC, and the book appeared in a number of newspapers and magazines over the course of the following month. What an adventure.

Since being published, the courage of the authors of the various chapters have been inspiring parents across the globe. Their willingness to be vulnerable in the hopes that sharing their stories would help someone else who had found themselves in a similar boat, has been enough to restore the hardest heart's faith in humanity, and the resulting book has been far more impacting than any of us ever could have imagined.

Needless to say, I am eternally grateful for each and every contributing author, but more than that, I am in absolute awe of their ability to rise above their own circumstances and give wholeheartedly to so many others. They are all amazing human beings and I am truly grateful to have been able to work with them.

After the launch and the excitement had passed, I thought that was the end of that particular story, and I threw myself into a number of new publishing projects.

Then the questions started coming...

- What had happened to all the authors?
- Did Cindy get her school started?
- Did Randa get her MATES program off the ground?
- What about the kids? What are they all doing now?

Finally, and quite organically, the idea was put forward that we put together a follow up book and lots of the authors agreed it was a great idea. They had experienced lots of change and growth in the years since they had written their first chapters and they were keen to write about the changes.

Introduction
by Deborah Fay

It has been so exciting to work with many of the authors once again. Every single one of them are doing amazing things and they are so good to work with. I think, in essence, we all want the same things – to feel connected, and to help others.

I know you will enjoy catching up with the authors and reading about what is happening in their lives now. One thing I can promise is that every single story you are about to read is an adventure and you will be at least as inspired by their journeys now as you were when you read their first stories.

Enjoy,

Deb x

DEBORAH FAY *is the Founder and CEO of Disruptive Publishing. Her commitment to publishing real stories by real people about topics that matter is evident in the type and number of books she has published to date. Deborah offers a range of coaching support and done-for-you services for aspiring authors.*

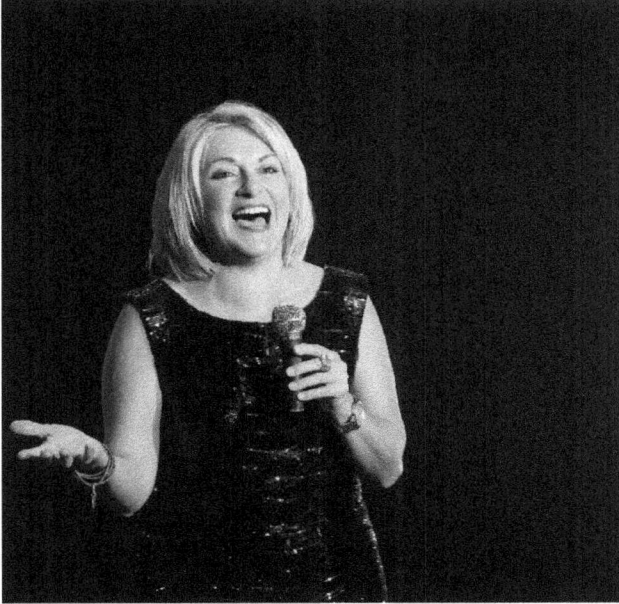

#ThomasKentCan
by Julie Cross

We had got to 14, and we were doing better... we were a family that not only had Autism along for the ride, but also the grief of me losing my husband, and my boys their dad, so the journey had definitely been more complicated. Grief is a tough taskmaster, but grief with Autism along for the ride is a whole new level. Daddy died, so in Thomas's world of concrete thinking, that Autism-world where it is difficult to abstract think and 'put it aside' and see through to the possibility that you can live around the grief – well, in his world it was always going to take a lot longer to learn how to process the grief and then move through it. So, if Daddy died, then when is mummy going to die? And when the grief was deep Autism got so loud. Perhaps you can relate.

So, considering all of that, we were through the worst of the smashed-up walls, the swearing, and then that stage where he used to call me a big penis all the time... I don't know why!? So, yes, we were through the worst of that and I did learn how to grow through moments like that. Oh, yes, Thomas did teach me so much about how to muscle up mentally so that the tough moments didn't break you; instead, you could see, with the benefit of looking back, that in fact those moments *made* you. So, when Thomas was calling me a 'big penis', I was thinking to myself... 'Well, I wouldn't mind one just quietly!' And so, I have a giggle to myself, taking pride in my ability to stay in touch with my sense of humour. And my energy lifts, my mood is better, and that has to be better for all of us, right?

And now here we are, further along the journey, and still we have some challenges – or moments that will grow us, which is how we look at it when we have the energy to take the positive stance. We have had some wins along the way too, and now I would love to share some more of that story with you.

Thomas did well in his high school years. No, he was not academically up with his peers, and we were lucky that the school Thomas attended had a great vocational program and that they recognised the need to celebrate all achievements, and not just those academically. Thomas did his Certificate 2 in Hospitality in his final two years of school, and he would work one day a week at The Coffee Club supported by an Agency – meaning he was given assistance at the coffee shop and this was all part of the 'funding' available, my first glimpse at a system that looks helpful on first contact but, I would discover further along the journey is not as helpful as they would like us to think – but more on that later.

Thomas has never stopped surprising me, and I don't ever want you to stop believing in the possibilities, the possibility of these young children growing and learning and reaching milestones every day. Celebrate progress, not perfection, and stop comparing progress – it will just deflate you and steal your joy. These children and adults on the spectrum really are here to challenge the way we see and acknowledge growth and potential, and what we 'think' and 'feel' is really important. And I truly believe that we as a society need to be challenged on all of that.

You know if you had asked me – his Mother, who is supposed to know him the best – what job Thomas would like to do at the Coffee Club, I would have said, "Out the back washing dishes, somewhere away from most of the people. After all, Autism isn't very social." Well, it turns out that Thomas loves all the people! Perhaps it is just me he doesn't like! Haha... but yes, he loved serving the customers, knew all their names and they knew his. Possibilities don't let us believe everything we read about how Autism looks and presents. Yes, they may be on the spectrum, but they are all still individuals and they all have the ability to grow and learn in their own time!

I remember at primary school telling the teachers to take 'Make eye contact' off his Individual Learning Program. I remember saying to them that we just had to let it go. Thomas will make eye contact when he is comfortable and ready. And who is 'making eye contact' really making feel better? And why? Because someone decided once that making eye contact is good manners? Please, just leave it alone.

And so, as I sit in the coffee shop observing Thomas at work, I watch him making eye contact with the customers. Yes, in his own time, he will rise to the occasion. I watched him walk up to a young couple sitting at a table. A man and woman... he walks towards them with two drinks on his tray. He makes eye contact and says, 'Iced coffee?' The young lady responds and says that it is hers. He puts it carefully in front of her. He then looks back at the couple, one drink on his tray and one man in front of him without a drink... but still he looks at the drink, back at the couple and says, 'Chocolate Milkshake?' The young man smiles, looks around, and then responds that it was his... Thomas carefully places the drink in front of him, tucks the tray under his arm and gives them 'The Wiggles' fingers as he says, 'Enjoy those drinks!'

As he walks away this young couple smile at him, they smile at each other and touch each other as they talk about Thomas in a warm and loving manner. Maybe they don't know why Thomas is different, maybe they can't quiet put their finger on it, but they know he is, and isn't that wonderful! You see, in my work I teach people on the so called 'Normal Spectrum' how to put more of 'them' into each customer service interaction so that you may surprise and delight your customers, giving them a unique experience; and here was my son, my son on the 'Autism Spectrum', doing just that.

You can have your OP1s – for this Mummy, that moment right there was equal to a university degree... all progress is celebrated. Thomas is a burst of colour in a world of beige, and I was seeing that really clearly now. It was a little blurry and hard to see when the walls and windows were being smashed in, so if that is where you are at, don't lose faith and hang in there.

When it comes to inclusion and celebrating and accommodating children of all different backgrounds and differing abilities, I think we are doing better in lots of schools, and for us it was a positive experience. However, I would discover that it was a different experience once Thomas finished school and was out in the world as an adult; that would be when I would realise that we truly don't get what inclusion really is about.

Let me explain...

There was a moment when our family went out for breakfast. My other son Jack and I got our breakfast and sat down, and Thomas got his and sat down... on another table! Now, my ego wanted to make him sit with us and be 'normal' so that we could get the perfect Instagram photo of this happy family, but what I have learnt is that true inclusion would mean that as his Mum, his leader, my job is not to make him fit in – my role is to give him a stage to feel safe, to feel validated for standing out and being who he is. That is true inclusion. We have so much to learn from how these children and adults see and process the world around them, and we will miss that learning while we are trying to make them fit in.

So, we finished school on a high! Thomas won awards... not of the academic kind, but the kind where you get rewarded for doing your best against the odds. We were so proud, and then hopeful that he would continue working at The Coffee Club.

I felt like I had let my breath out and relaxed, we had got through school we had made it. But then, as I allowed myself to celebrate that we had got here, we had done it... well, it was just after that I took a sharp breath back in and held it. He didn't get the job at The Coffee Club; you see, they would take on another young person doing a course and while giving them experience they effectively get two employees (the student and an assistant) with no monetary commitment from the workplace, as it is funded. So, the cracks start to appear in the system, and I realise that the journey hasn't finished – it has just begun. We are back at the pre-school of adulthood and I would have to facilitate that journey every step of the way... and if not me, then whom?

Now, I did allow myself the reflection and the celebration, but then I realised very quickly that employers still really have no idea what Autism is and what the benefits are of having someone in the team on the spectrum, and so in reality in this country there is a very low rate of adults with Autism that gain employment. I am suddenly trying to learn about a system that promised us support gaining employment and yet I felt the doors shut at every turn. And you see, I don't understand a system where I must scream out about what Thomas can't do to get attention and get assistance... all we wanted was for Thomas to get a job... a hand-up, not a hand-out. But I don't want this story to be about everything that is wrong, I don't want this to be about what we still are not doing to demonstrate and embrace true inclusion and embracing diversity. I do want this to be about having hope; not giving up, and in doing so educating a community about the value that Autism brings to the world around them.

The first year out of school Thomas got his licence. He was on his learner's permit while at school and we were slowly building up those 100 hours. I initially started out feeling nervous about Thomas driving, but quickly realised that

Thomas was going to be a great driver. Of course, he is, he is a rule follower and has a great memory. So, he quickly picked it up, and not once was there ever a discussion about whether he should or shouldn't get his licence, if he was capable; of course, he should. Independence is the greatest gift that I can give Thomas, and he has been very self-sufficient from a young age. Our family heartache – my husband having a stroke and me being a busy single mum with two boys, one with Autism – meant that I didn't have the time and space to be overprotective: no helicopter parenting here. It is not a style for the feint hearted, and I admit that the first time he got a train to the shops, well I drove beside the train the whole way. But I couldn't do that every time, so I had to faith it until we made it, and Thomas would show me that he would have much better problem-solving skills than we ever gave him credit for. And in fact, he would develop some of that abstract thinking that that children on the spectrum seem to be challenged with. In reflection, how on earth can our kids learn problem-solving skills if they are never allowed to face a problem on their own? As I said, not for the feint hearted, but for us it was a blessing in disguise, because Thomas grew in ways I couldn't have imagined.

So, the day he got his P's and passed that driving test, well – the whole family dissolved into tears. Tears of relief, of accomplishment of belief, of disbelief... another important milestone reached, and I watched Thomas grow taller with a confidence that can only come through personal achievement. We were all so proud of him, and yet again I needed nerves of steel watching him drive away in the car on his own. I wanted to put wheel locks on his car with a sign that said, 'Ask Mummy if you can go out and drive the car' just like we used to do with his bike when he was little. But no, this is what we have been working towards; now, Mummy, practice trust and faith. And so, we did, and we do.

Thomas then did another Certificate in Hospitality and I was still trying to work out how the 'system' was supporting my son to find a job, because we actually do get that promise. I mean, we talk inclusion all the time, don't we?

Thomas would go to many interviews. I was mystified again about how the system works and wondering who was advocating for Thomas, who was explaining to employees that Thomas may not present well in an interview due to his inability to communicate directly when put in a stressful situation. I mean, he was competing with young people on the 'normal spectrum' – there was no sign on his forehead saying he was Autistic and had communication issues, but that he would be an honest, loyal and committed employee, that he would need to be shown what was expected but that once he learnt the skills of the job he would do them perfectly every time, that when you hire Thomas you would be getting somebody that would never try to shirk his responsibilities or avoid the mundane jobs... so who is doing that for Thomas? Well, the truth is that nobody could answer that for me.

Thomas would keep saying to me, 'Mum, when am I getting a job?' 'Mum, I need to earn money...' So, here is a young man that just wants to work. He needs a purpose and a reason to get up every morning, just like we all do.

I am not going to go into the NDIS system, one I haven't yet negotiated, but any system that requires for me to be 'in the right head space' just to start the process due to the frustration of the process... well, I would say the system needs work. And I will not focus on what Thomas CANNOT do; instead, I will make that the focus on our conversations, whether they be with friends, families or people in official capacities making judgements on what they think Thomas needs. I just knew he needed a job, and he will grow and develop in all kinds of ways through having one!

So, with the growing frustration of nothing happening in the job front, I could feel Thomas's mood and energy change; I could feel him becoming frustrated and a little angry, which of course was mostly directed at me. It was time to make something happen, and if I don't who will?

It was the middle of the night and I suddenly had a thought... everybody focuses on what Autism can't do, what about everything Thomas CAN do? And maybe I feel a little responsible for that, I did share our journey of wall smashing, window breaking, swearing and spitting very openly, and I did it for all the right reasons. To make others feel less alone, to be open and honest and vulnerable about how big this journey really is, but now is that all people were seeing? You see, Thomas does not smash walls and windows anymore, Thomas is polite and caring and loves to please and treat people with respect. Thomas is social, and hell, he can even look people in the eye! Just like everybody else, Thomas can grow and learn, and he has!

We started collecting cans for cash. He got some friends collecting them, and he would take them to the recycle place and get his 10 cents a can. At the beginning I would go with him, and then he would do it independently. Just in doing this I could see him feel good, feel good about doing something himself and getting paid. And for me it is about being prepared to do what it takes and starting from the beginning. But we needed to do more, and I was getting tired of people asking, 'What would Thomas like to do?' How they hell do we know yet? You are asking the wrong question – it is not what he would like to do, it is about what we are prepared to do. And I believe that is the question to be asking all young people getting started.

Yes, it is time to start talking about what Thomas CAN DO, and what he is prepared to do. Let's stop waiting for something to happen and *make* something happen. And this was the beginning of a business idea – 'Thomas Kent Can' – so we got him an ABN and insurance, set up a Facebook page and started a business. Thomas Kent can clean windows, clean cars, mow lawns, wash dogs, walk dogs, watch dogs – yes, Thomas Kent Can!

We launched the business and as I write this, we are three weeks in. I have been going to a lot of the jobs with him, so as I find myself in 30-degree heat Googling how to start a Honda whipper snipper, I say to myself, 'How the hell did I get here?' But of course, I wouldn't change a thing. We have been walking and washing dogs, cleaning houses and cars. We will work out what he can do without me and we aim to get regular jobs and customers, so that he can do his jobs without me present. He has been earning about $450 a week so far. Now, the $450 is nice and it sure helps, but what it is really about is seeing his growth. I have been blown away seeing his communication skills develop, his confidence skyrocket, his organisational skills grow, and his self-esteem strengthen... and that is what this is really all about!

I have no clue where this will all lead, and I don't need to know that – just progress, and one day at a time. I feel I have a mission to educate the world now about the gifts that Autism brings to a workforce, because, you see, not every parent can go and start a business for their children... and the reason we do that is because nobody will give them a job, so that is the real problem.

In a world full of beige, in a time where businesses are filled with people delivering habitual and routine service, in a time when we are shouting out for people to be unique and stand out for the crowd rather than blend in... well it seems to me that there is no better time for our children to shine. Let us be truly inclusive and embrace the gifts that Autism brings and stop trying to make them fit in, but instead give them a stage to stand out on.

We will all benefit from that!

*Meet **JULIE CROSS** – a mother, author and, well, some people say one of the most inspiring keynote speakers in Australia. She combines incredible insights into human behaviour with practical strategies that leave her audiences with powerful tools for living their best life and setting a higher standard in all aspects of their existence.*

Affectionately known as 'sparkles', Julie is not just a high energy speaker with a few shiny sound bites. She is able to connect her message of inspiration, motivation and practical personal development at all levels of business – from corporate CEOs to mothers, fathers and teenagers, and everybody in between.

But... her proudest achievement is being a mother of two boys, one living with Autism and all the challenges and triumphs that come from that and one living with being typical... and all the triumphs and challenges that come with that!

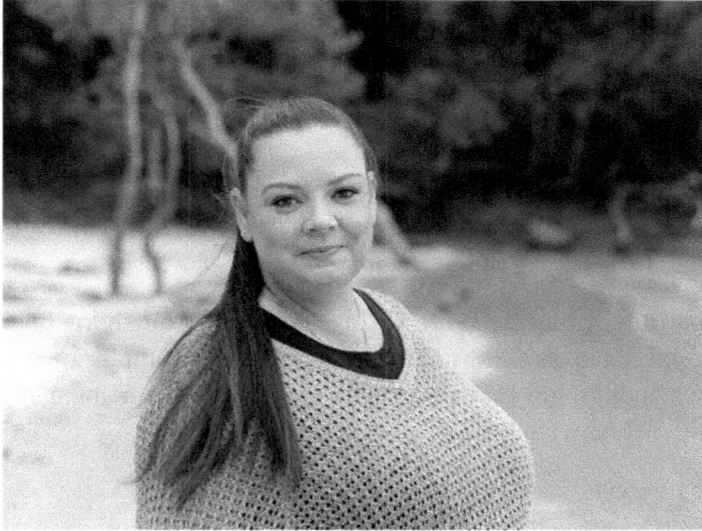

Kindness Empowers
by Letisha Living

CHILD ONE

Oh wow, what a journey this is!

I remember where we were five or so years ago, and I am so relieved that those days of battling it out in the Family Law Courts for an Order to undertake assessments, diagnosis and interventions for my child are well and truly behind us. I would love to say that things got resolved as time went by, but my greater family dynamics remain dysfunctional.

I have learned through these experiences how to respond better when life throws me a curve ball.

One of the biggest takeaways on reflection of where things were for me when the first *Parenting A Child On The Spectrum* book was published is that it is so important to trust your instincts, continue to be that voice and advocate for your children's wellbeing.

That situation has not changed for me at all, some days I still feel like I am a lonely voice speaking up, raising my hand, waving my arms, wanting to be heard and validated for the sake of my children.

Note: I may intermittently refer to my 'children' from here on instead of referring to my 'child' as I now have two children with complex needs (since the last book was published) that I am single parenting, plus being a young stroke survivor with my own challenges.

Ahh, that curveball.

The child that I wrote about when the first book was published was in his early primary school years at that time. He has now commenced his high school adventures.

A year ago, I was feeling upset with the inclusion in mainstream system. I appreciate that there are adjustments to the curriculum to accommodate my child's differences, however, we were having the same ongoing difficulties.

I had wondered whether home-schooling would be a better learning environment for my son. At school he was displaying extreme anxiety and I felt he was missing out on too many lunch breaks. He was internalising messages that he was inherently bad and not able to make correct choices.

From my perspective, when you get an educator for your child who can see your child's behaviours as a way of communication, has the insight to re-direct before behaviour escalates, builds a trusting relationship with them, has open communication with you and will take on board your suggestions to help, it is like winning the lotto.

On the flip side, I found that when you get an educator whose personality is prejudiced, that impact was insidious – not just to my child, but to our whole family unit.

As previously mentioned, my son has now commenced high school. This transition has been better than I could have ever imagined.

The high school has a special education department, with specialised teaching staff who are open and understanding.

It has been such a relief! The communication has been amazing.

Last year, I was spending most days in tears at the thought of sending my child to school. This year I am spending most days shedding tears of relief that he is okay and actually wants to go to school.

CHILD TWO

I would love to say that I am so glad that the battle for a diagnosis or approval for government funding are over for us, but I cannot, as this continues through my youngest child who has a severe developmental delay.

This time around the ongoing struggle to move forward is not with family members, but with the support agencies that conduct the assessments and make the decisions for diagnosis and funding.

The assessments that the clinics and support agencies undertake have reported severe findings, however my child remains in the void of not eligible for a diagnosis or funding, despite needing (requiring) a lot of ongoing therapies.

I could probably write another book on this experience, too!

I have learned to accept that I will be challenged by the very people who I think are supposed to help me and be on my team.

Some people won't see what I see, because they are not living my life, or they just don't have that insight and understanding about my children and my family dynamic as I do.

There have been many times when I have felt all alone in this world and I wondered why I was given this task of raising children with complex needs. Especially when I have my own challenges resulting from my stroke.

THE JUDGEMENTS OF OTHERS

I wake every morning knowing in my heart that I just want to do what's best for my children, that I might not get it right and that when they close their eyes each night, that they know that they are loved, safe and whole just as they are, no matter what happened during that day.

When I have an overwhelming moment (e.g. I yell at them), I make a conscious effort to apologise to them so that they know that their behaviour is not bad and that I am not perfect either.

There have been many times where I have had to put on my biggest, bravest 'pretend I am okay' face in public and then collapse into tears later on when no one is around.

There have been countless moments of heartbreak as I have watched those closest to us and/or complete strangers judge my children's meltdowns, unusual behaviours or my parenting of them.

It is so upsetting to watch your child grow up being excluded from social play and birthday parties.

The comments below are some of the things that have been said directly to me over the years as my children have been growing up. Some of them had me doubting myself over and over. I wonder who else can relate to some of these?

I hope that I am not alone in having had some of these divisive thoughts projected on to me.

- If he were my kid, this is how I would do it differently;
- If he's hungry enough, he will eat it;
- Why are you giving him a choice, just tell him this is how it is;
- He is 'choosing' to behave this way (during full scale meltdown);
- We think you are enabling him;
- He is old enough to know better;
- He is just being a brat;
- You must have done something when you were pregnant;
- Vaccination causes that;
- Do you receive government money because he has that?;
- I read on XYZ website that it can be cured by XYZ;
- Take away his favourite thing and give him a good smack, that's what worked when I was growing up;
- That's not typical of ASD, I know of another child who has ASD, and they are totally differently to what you're saying right now;
- You should put him on medication;
- Why aren't you medicating him yet?;
- What usually happens with ASD is...;
- He's not talking because everyone else is doing the talking for him;
- He's just being rude and disrespectful;
- He seems normal to me;
- Ohhh, you poor thing;
- Why haven't you told him what's wrong with him yet;
- Just ignore him and he will stop doing it;
- He will grow out of it;
- Why is he still doing that? You've told him so many times not to do that;
- People are just after a diagnosis for everything these days;

- (Statistically) What we have seen is children who make poor behaviour choices tend to have poorer outcomes in high school and in life;

and

- He is X years old; he should know better by now.

Sometimes it isn't just what a person *says* that can be soul crushing; sometimes it is the complete lack of empathy and interpersonal connection, the zero-verbal response when there should be one, the blank facial expressions and closed body language that hurts the most.

Sometimes the most pain is felt by all of the things these people aren't *saying* or *doing*, but their *judgement* and *invalidation* is coming across loud and clear.

Before parenting children with complex needs, I have wondered if I was just as unaware and hurtful as some of these people who have said these comments to me.

I have certainly learned how to have a thicker skin and understand that what comes out of other people's mouths reflects where their mindsets are, and those beliefs are not a reflection of me or my children.

Despite being a young stroke survivor with my own challenges and single parenting two special needs children, this journey has been far from only stressful.

I am so thankful to say that I feel like the days of despair are behind us.

I still have some not so good days every now and then.

I still question myself and wonder if I am getting it right.

I still read all about Autism Spectrum Disorders and attend professional seminars. One of my highlights of 2019 was having a 1:1 conversation and taking a selfie with Professor Tony Attwood.

I do feel like I have been given these children to teach me how to become a better person. My life feels so much richer and fuller for letting them teach me how to do life differently. We have certainly moved away from whatever is conditioned societal norms and we much prefer to do life on our terms.

I no longer waste my time or energy trying to convince closed minded people to see things from another perspective if they are not open or receptive to change.

I no longer seek others' approval of us.

I no longer try to justify myself or my children's behaviour to others.

I no longer make my children apologise for melting down (or shutting down) to an adult who refused to accommodate to their sensory (or other) needs which caused the meltdown to occur in the first place.

My children do think and act differently to what society defines as 'neurotypical' and I love that the most about them.

My children challenge the status-quo, allow me to have deeper human experiences and to love unconditionally.

They aren't always in meltdown mode, destroying things, running around in circles flapping their hands and refusing to speak, eat or sleep.

They aren't always in front of a screen either.

When life isn't overwhelming them (or me), they are the kindest, most caring and funniest kids to be around. Sometimes we even get out of our pyjamas and leave the house, ha-ha.

KINDNESS EMPOWERS

My children want the exact same things in life that anyone else wants, and that is to be accepted for who they are, to feel a sense of belonging, to be loved unconditionally and to be treated with Kindness.

It has been through this life experience and parenting these children that I have learned that *Kindness Empowers*.

It has been incredibly life changing for me to receive acts of Kindness from others. Simple things like a smile from another person when I am having a hard day, someone listening to me without judgement, showing compassion for my children, being heard and valued, including and accommodating the needs of my children without me having to fight for it have left a profound impact on me.

Kindness has let me know that I am not alone in this world. My quirky, unique and unconventional family dynamic is okay.

That we are okay just the way we are.

That we all deserve to be respected and loved for who we are and not forced to become a by-product of someone else's expectations of us.

In September 2019, through my business lawyer, I trademarked the words 'Kindness Empowers'.

It has become my mission to spread ripples (tidal waves) of Kindness out into the world to empower others, turn their unique inner light on, allow them to shine brighter and let people know that they are never alone.

We connect and achieve more together through kindness.

If you are having a hard day, feeling all beat up, unheard, overwhelmed or exhausted, I want you to know that you are not alone, you are amazing, and you are doing a great job.

I see you.

I feel you.

I hear you.

Your presence matters.

#KindnessEmpowers

LETISHA LIVING *is a young stroke survivor and mum of four boys. It is her youngest two sons who present with complex needs.*

It has been through this journey of life and parenting that inspired Letisha to create the #KindnessEmpowers effect.

Letisha enjoys reiki & meditation, being outdoors and spending quality time with friends and family.

Follow her messages of kindness and inspiration on Instagram @FreeBirdsLiving

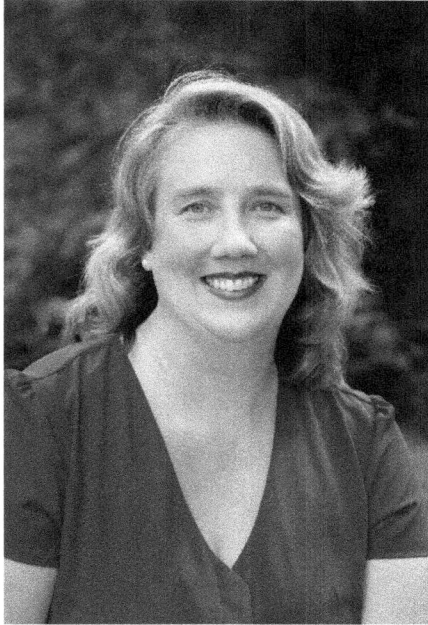

Double Dipper – the Ride of a Lifetime with Two
by Catherine Rosalion

SCHOOL TO HOME

Educating a child on the spectrum, like everything else, is a bumpy ride. Soon after naming my first child, Sebastian, my next biggest decision was where he'd go to school. I thought I had it all planned out from kinder to high school when I stumbled across the Montessori system while chatting to mums at a breastfeeding group. Kinder went surprisingly well. Sebastian had two of the most caring and dynamic teachers I could ever wish for, who accepted and loved him as he was. They were able to channel his obsessions with maths, washing dishes and flags to learning in other areas. They cherished his quirkiness and found creative solutions (such as them wearing headphones) for his never-ending monologue.

Sebastian transitioned relatively easily into school, but then the roller-coaster slowly began to derail. Three years with the same teacher (as is the way in the Montessori system) had lulled us into a false sense of security. His little safety bubble burst with a teacher and peer-group change. By the start of grade 5 all his friends, including his best mate, had moved onto high school (being gifted, he always socialised with much older children). I never understood the challenge parents faced when their child was 'school refusing'. I thought (but never said), 'Just get them in the car and take them to school for goodness' sake!' Oh, my naivety! This was now my life.

Over the school holidays, my son's anxiety skyrocketed. Not knowing how he'd cope making new friends was just too much to think about, and he started to withdraw. By the time grade five started, he had made up a story in his head that it was going to be intolerable without his best friend, and he didn't want to go. I had a child who was 11 years old, wearing size small men's clothing with feet bigger than mine, who refused to get out of bed. Even on the days when I could physically get him out of bed, a process which could take hours, he would then retreat to the lounge-room and roll himself up in the rug like a burrito. Attempting to coax him to put on his uniform or get into the car were more impossible battles I was never going to win. We struggled to attain a half time attendance record for term one, which then became zero attendance by term two. The school did nothing to help, and there was not a single friend who understood our struggles. Friends were saying to me, 'Just be tough and tell him he has to go to school!' or 'Bribe him with more screen time.' (The latter I had actually tried, despite how I despise bribery, but it hadn't worked!) Much to my horror, the mother of his best mate threatened that he wouldn't be allowed to play computer games with her son if he didn't go to school. This scared him enough to get out of bed and half put on his uniform the next day, but then he ran to the toilet and sat huddled on the floor with crippling tummy pains from anxiety, eventually retreating to the rug where he slept the rest of the day.

With our social worker, occupational therapist (OT) and psychologist on board, I arranged meetings with the school, but nothing was working to get him back. He was far too disengaged. So began our search for another school. I had interviews and tours of all the local, and not so local, government schools, and while Sebastian turned his nose up at all of them, many of the principals told us their school may not work for him anyway given the Montessori pedagogy he was used to. We stumbled across an alternative independent school that funnily enough was the first option I considered years earlier, and Sebastian fell back in love with learning. This exuberance was short lived (as I had feared), and as making new friends became challenging, and not wanting to sleep over at school camp set him apart as 'different', and he was school refusing again. This time, however, the school was amazing. The first day he missed a day of school I had phone calls from his teacher, the secretary and principal, all asking what they could do to help get him back. The day he returned to school I will never forget the sight I saw out my window as I drove off. His teacher bounded through the classroom door and ran across the muddy grass field towards him with open arms (like the first scene in 'The Sound of Music') and held him in a tight embrace. Wow! If only all schools were like this one.

Despite all this effort from the school, and his psychologist, Sebastian withdrew rapidly. I resigned myself to the fact we were destined to home school and boarded a new rollercoaster, one I wished in hindsight I started so much earlier. As a teacher myself, the logical thing would have been for me to take over his education, but he was a pre-teen with ASD and a myriad of other issues. I could hardly get him to pick up his dirty socks off the floor, let alone 'teach' him. Instead, I was now his personal assistant. I advertised for tutors, enrolled him in classes, madly caught up to speed on the current state educational standards, and became his chauffeur. He had a secondary school science and cooking teacher extraordinaire tutoring him at home, every week did group tennis coaching, individual art and drum lessons, maths and science gifted classes, a gifted day school program (that meant 4 hours of driving for me!), advanced maths tutoring, weekly psychology, fortnightly social group and monthly OT. It's exhausting just writing it all down! This term sent me completely broke, and I still had not paid off the previous term of private schooling. It was financially the hardest time we had ever experienced as a family, and without the amazing support in the community (just to be able to eat), we would not have survived.

TWO BECAME FOUR

During these years, it was not only the turmoil with school that Sebastian had been dealing with. It had only been Sebastian and I for eight years, so his world came crashing down when I braved the online dating world and thought I had finally found 'the one'. After weeks of chatting, our first date was at a play centre and he gifted Sebastian an encyclopaedia on gemstones. He had asked about his Autism and remembered what his current obsession was, wow!

This relationship that started off so perfectly (in my eyes!) began to rapidly unravel. It became really challenging for an outsider to understand parenting a child on the spectrum, and all the other complications, like sensory issues and anxiety, that come with the territory. I had this Autism parenting gig down to a fine art, and it wasn't that I knew what I was doing necessarily, nor that how I did things was the right or only way – but it was our way, and it was working (mostly!). If nothing else, I was the specialist on my child and knew him better than anyone. My new partner trying to make changes wasn't helping any of us. His resentment soon turned into anger, with him yelling and using verbal and emotional abuse to manipulate both of us.

I went to see a psychologist thinking I was going insane (well, more crazy than I already was after years of single-parenting a child with special needs) and she warned me that there were so many red flags I needed to get out *now*. My partner convinced me that it was indeed the psychologist who was nuts and stopped me from going to see her anymore. A long trip overseas early in our relationship seemed to make my heart grow fonder, and the time apart helped me distance myself and forget all the trauma. I came home longing to have another child with him and got pregnant as quickly the second time as I did the first (despite being told by professionals it could take years!).

Despite desperately wanting to have this child, I was still not ready to move in together. I went through the whole pregnancy on my own which was immensely challenging. I had a great deal of pelvic pain and had to stop work as I could hardly walk, let alone get up and down off the floor with the kids with ASD I was working with. Not to mention, I still had my own child on the spectrum to parent. While we were meant to be in the honeymoon stage of our relationship, and attempting to plan for parenting together, we could not agree on anything. How was this ever going to work?

My family of two soon became four. I finally got to have the water birth I'd always dreamed of, and my gorgeous daughter Ava (the only name that came close to a three-way compromise) entered our world. She came so quickly the birthing pool was only half full, and she stole our hearts just as fast. The day of her birth was just as blissful as our first date. Although, this blur could have been all the oxytocin and severe sleep deprivation! I thought I could never love anyone as much as I loved my son, but it seemed I still had more love to give. I sat there embracing my baby, tears of joy rolling down my cheeks splashing softly into the water. In the eerie silence, there was a brief moment when the nurse realised my baby was blue and not breathing as she had her cord wrapped around her neck. She was wrenched out of my arms, but the second she was lifted up a cry resounded throughout the room and we were reunited.

Some measly hours after giving birth, I discharged myself from the sterile hospital to the comfort of my own home and for the next two weeks, life seemed perfect. My partner brought me freshly squeezed orange juice in bed every morning and delivered me glasses of water every time I needed to breastfeed (which was pretty constant, and I felt like a 24/7 milk bar!). Ava seemed calm and settled as long as she was held but putting her down even for a moment didn't work, as she screamed like her bassinette was on fire. The baby-wearing and co-sleeping I had planned for, that my partner never wanted, became a necessity.

FEAR TO FEEDOM

The newborn baby bliss abruptly came to an end after only a fortnight. There was only so long my partner could hold in his rage, and I had post-natal depression (again), not surprising given the strongest preventative factor is having a supportive partner. I had always wondered if becoming a parent himself would make him more understanding and loving towards my son, but alas, the opposite occurred. Sebastian became a second-class citizen to his new sister.

Sebastian has huge sensory issues as part of his Autism, and one of them is how defensive he is to loud noises. I bought him noise cancelling headphones very early in his life when shopping centres and birthday parties were too overwhelming. So, when my previously quiet and placid baby started to scream continuously and hardly slept, Sebastian couldn't cope. One day, the crying was so intense that Sebastian ran to his room to hide in his bed, slamming his door behind him. My partner flew into a furious rage and stormed into Sebastian's room so quickly after him that he smashed Sebastian behind his own door, pushing him against the wall, cutting his toe and scaring him senseless as he screamed a tornado of abuse. Once I could get into his room, I found a pale, shivering child huddled behind the door, soaked in his own tears and urine. I held him so tight and we sobbed together, and all I could say was 'sorry' over and over again. I called the police, who I thought would help, but my 'Jekyll and Hyde' partner managed to convince them he was an angel. I took both my kids in my arms and left my home barefoot, but where could we go? Although I had broken up the relationship and tried to leave many times before, this was the moment I realised I had left it way too late. I was no novice either, as I had left previous partners, including when I was pregnant with Sebastian because of the bruises and abuse. Why didn't I know better, and why was it so hard to leave?

For whatever reason, the countless apologies and the gifts of Lego to try and buy back Sebastian's trust seemed enough for us to attempt to stay yet again. Five months later, when we were being evicted from our rental property of 8 years, I told my partner that this was the end! When the movers came, we were going our separate ways. He went silent and stormed out of the house, as he did whenever he didn't get his way, and vanished for the day. I got the usual text messages from him claiming to be intoxicated (although he never drank), threatening to kidnap my daughter or commit suicide if I left him. Eventually he came home but was in a scary and distant mood. He snatched Ava out of my arms and took her to our bedroom. As Ava hollered every time anyone other than me held her, she was hysterical. I was too terrified to open the door and retrieve my screaming baby, as the phone helpline counsellor warned me not to interfere and reminded me of the case where the angry father killed his daughter throwing her off a bridge. I sat helplessly in the garden in the dark, clenching my knees and rocking back and forth, not unlike a depiction of the early visions of children with Autism. It was my son who was brave enough to go into that bedroom and tell my partner to give the baby back to me. To this day I am in awe of his bravery, and how he stands up for, and protects, his sister.

Once I had Ava safely back in my arms, I gazed into her tear stained face, red and purple with broken capillaries around her eyes. I immediately called the police, but again they were of no help. They couldn't get him to leave, even though it was my name on the lease and I was paying all the rent! I whispered to my son to go and pack a bag of clothes and nappies, and the second my partner stepped foot in the shower we escaped. I had been unable to take my baby out in the car at all, as she would scream to the point of turning blue and vomiting on herself, but now my only choices were to be housebound with an abusive partner, or drive with my baby in a sling to a friend's house for refuge. What would you do? After a sleepless night, I dropped Sebastian at his safe haven of school, and returned home to meet the moving truck. My manipulative ex had deliberately not labelled his boxes, so the movers had to move everything together and again he came with us.

Living 'separated under one roof' was meant to be for a few days while we sorted out belongings, but we struggled on until Ava turned one. Her early development was delayed but the maternal child health nurse kept urging us to wait and see. She was hardly crawling, had many words but wouldn't use them, still didn't sleep for longer than an hour, had severe sensory issues, and didn't really 'play'. She also had profound separation anxiety and had to be held by me 24/7. The only other person she had a special bond with was her brother, as they just seemed to get each other.

One night, I went out with my kids to my choir Christmas party (in a taxi of course!) and answered a desperate call from a friend who needed to stay the night. She was escaping from her abusive partner, and our lives shared so many similarities. We met when both our Sebastians were babies (born only a few days apart), and years later we, and our sons, had become best of friends. We shared our struggles as both Sebastians were on the spectrum. We chatted every week while the boys attended Lego club, and at the same moment announced to each other over an iced chai that we were pregnant again (due days apart, of course!).

It was having another adult in the house, seeing and hearing what we were enduring, that convinced me that we had to get free. It took many weeks to formulate an escape plan with help from a domestic violence service, police and the court but finally when he left for work, all 6 of us – two single mums with our just-turned-one-year-olds and our sons with ASD – left. With an intervention order served, the police finally helped by removing my ex from our home while we stayed with friends. The locks were changed, cameras were installed, and it was safe enough (physically) to move back home.

Finally, we were free!

DOUBLE DIAGNOSES

With the freedom from abuse came a sudden surge in both kids development. Sebastian's anxiety lessened, he became more independent and started to come back out of his shell. He was even getting himself up and dressed each morning and walking himself to school. Ava no longer had to be vegan as my ex had insisted, so her gut issues and iron levels slowly improved, and she quickly began to use her words and finally walk. Her anxiety, however, did not disappear, and her quirky behaviours became more noticeable. She was very set in her routines (like having vitamins in the same order and only in her brother's bathroom), had huge tactile and auditory sensory issues (couldn't tolerate light touch or certain clothes), would 'play' by lining up dolls or puzzle pieces across the room, had strange fascinations with objects (like holding onto a rock to shower and sleep), had become an incredibly picky eater with a predominately 'white' diet, and did not seem to understand how to interact with others (yes, she was only one, but other kids would wave and say 'hi' and 'bye'. Still to this day she will not say 'good-bye'!).

Real-estate agents seem to think I revel in the idea of relocating with a baby, so once again we were evicted. I thought after moving we would all feel safer and these routines and behaviours which I was told Ava did to make her feel secure would vanish. My 11-year-old, however, seemed to become a moody, hormonal teenager overnight and I now had a tenacious toddler *and* a teen! Clearly, I did not think that one through!

We needed help! Sebastian was refusing to go to school, which soon morphed into refusing to go anywhere and just sleeping and reading his life away in his bedroom. We tried for half the year to get him to see a male psychologist who specialised in trauma but couldn't even get him out of the car. I found a brilliant psychologist who was recommended by another mum, and Sebastian began therapy. Granted there were some days it still took hours of arguing to get him into the car, but while Ava and I were upstairs in the waiting room, he would eventually appear in his own time. It took an hour a week for the entire term to complete his assessments, followed by another term of questionnaires going back and forth from two schools and multiple tutors.

At the end of Sebastian's assessment, I was lumped with a 30-page report, and he suddenly had a total of SIX diagnosis! Along with ASD, he now also had GAD (generalised anxiety disorder), depression, ADHD (attention deficit hyperactivity disorder), PDA (pervasive demand avoidance), and executive function disorder. He also had his giftedness confirmed (again), which came with another label, 'twice exceptional' (2e). None of these were a surprise but having them in writing would hopefully help us get the funding and help that he desperately needed. The paediatrician prescribed medication, but I never filled a script as every time he would refuse to eat thinking I had spiked his food. He was instantly granted a disability parking permit due to his high anxiety and aggressive outbursts that make going out anywhere next to impossible, and he would hopefully be reconsidered for the funding he was previously denied. Since his brief early intervention Autism package at age 6, Sebastian had no funding. I was told previously that as Sebastian was able to talk and not in nappies, he was not 'severe enough' to qualify for a companion card. If these people had lived a day with my child, they may have thought otherwise! It seemed even really close friends who had known my son for over 10 years could not fathom he had any challenges, and I was asked one day 'Why do you have a carers card?' then told, 'Wow that's insane, you don't have a child with a disability and now you can never work again, claim to have to care for your child, and sponge off the government!'

Simultaneously, because doing assessments with one child clearly was not enough of a challenge (physically, financially and emotionally), I sought to have Ava assessed. Our brilliant psychologist wanted to wait five years as kids with post-traumatic stress disorder (PTSD) following trauma can appear to have Autism. I Google researched like crazy and it seemed she was right, but I still wasn't convinced. Why would my child refusing to wear any clothes that were not pink or only eating pink food (this was a welcome addition to her otherwise 'white' diet) help her to feel safe? I could kind of see some logic behind liking order and routine, lining things up obsessively, and waking every hour all night long to check if I was still there.

My attempts at seeing another psychologist failed miserably, as call after call I was told that they would not diagnose a girl who was verbal so early and wanted to wait. Regardless of whether her issues were due to trauma or something else, the professional's opinion was that therapy would be the same, and she didn't need a diagnosis for early intervention funding, so why bother? Still fighting for answers, I put her on wait lists for services (déjà vu from years ago with Sebastian) and eventually Ava saw two paediatricians, another psychologist, a speech pathologist, had two hearing tests, and was already seeing an OT due to her sensory issues. Ava was selectively mute and would not interact with strangers, making the whole assessment process interesting to say the least. These professionals all unanimously agreed that Ava had ASD. Now I had two!

This time, being told I had a child on the spectrum did not come with the same relief as I was still confused. Being a girl, Ava seemed to present very differently to Sebastian with her Autism. I had read list upon list of signs of Autism in girls before seeking a diagnosis and she ticked every single box, but was it truly ASD or the result of trauma? I came out from the feedback session and messaged a friend to say, 'So I officially have two kids with ASD!'. Her reply will stay with me forever. She said, 'Great! You officially have two 'ausome' neuro-diverse kids who will make their mark on the world in their own unique way. Congratulations.' This was not something I thought was 'great' let alone deserved congratulations for, but I loved her positive outlook and have tried to embrace this ever since.

FIGHTING

I feel like I have spent my children's entire lives fighting for them, and what they needed and deserved. Getting the assessments done gave a formal indication of their strengths and areas where they needed help, but it was not going to guarantee access to funding, services, kinder or school. Having two kids with ASD and a trauma background meant that accessing specialist services was challenging. I had to fight to keep the professionals and services that I felt we needed in place when they claimed to not understand either Autism or DV. Ava was expelled from a child-care service that catered for women from DV relationships as 'she was too challenging and could not be settled'. When I asked to see their paperwork, I noticed they had a shocking clause about refusing to care for children with ASD and special needs. She later attempted an early kinder program, but again couldn't separate or settle for the two hours like the other children. This time I pulled her out, following the recommendation of the psychologist. We then spent 18 months on a waitlist for another kinder, but no matter how many phone calls, letters and emails I sent, I could not get her in. As a last resort, I asked the psychologist to write them a letter and within an hour of that being sent, I had an enrolment offer waiting in my inbox!

Given Sebastian had been out of the formal education system for most of the year and needed his peers, and home schooling was spiralling us more and more into debt, I applied for early entry into high school. To my amazement he got a letter of acceptance to the school of our choice. That was almost too easy! He was so excited he immediately called his friends and shouted his good news down the phone. He astonishingly completed his own enrolment forms and subject selections online.

Three months later, friends who also got in had been sent dates for parent information evenings and student orientation, which we hadn't received, so I made contact with the school. I am still in utter disbelief about what happened next. I was told Sebastian's enrolment was conditional upon receiving his full psychological report (which at this stage we didn't have) to prove he had a high IQ and was 12 months ahead, and his enrolment offer was rescinded. This rejection letter, coincidentally, was received a day after the cut-off date for making an appeal! If I had not already sought this assessment for Sebastian, then how would I miraculously make this happen with months waiting to get into the psychologist, not to mention the months it took for assessments and report? This rejection plummeted Sebastian further into depression and heighted his anxiety. Did the school realise or care what their decision was doing to my son?

I spent hours of my time and mental energy fighting for my son, for his right to have an education and to be considered for a place at a school like his peers, who did not need to submit psychological assessments. I did an internal appeal with the school and this was rejected. I then appealed through the Department of Education, writing a 10-page letter detailing why my son needed to be at this school, and supplied letters from both tutors and psychologists, but this appeal was also declined. I was told I had no more avenues of appeal but was not ready to stop fighting. I kept calling and emailing the department to no avail. After sending his now completed report directly to the school we were offered an interview with the principal. We both finally saw a glimmer of hope. At the interview he started by asking the usual questions like 'What subjects do you like?' but moved to interrogating him about why he had a fear of strangers, felt a need to keep weapons by his bed, and how he would cope around lots of people with his sensory issues. I sat in the room biting my tongue letting my son answer these questions on his own and despite his flat affect, I thought he was rather eloquent. We were told the Montessori program at the school was full. Well no kidding! After changing their minds about his enrolment, they had offered him the interview the day after the orientation program.

The next letter I received from the principal shocked and saddened me. I finally found out the real reason they did not want my son at their school was because of his special needs. They claimed they 'will not support the recommendations in his report' and suggested 'he can only be supported in a therapeutic setting'. Surely this was discrimination? I got on my high horse and called the Association for Children with a Disability (ACD) and sought legal help. The following day, I had my case ready to appeal through the department yet again. If he was refused enrolment because we lived out the zone or because of his young age, fine, I couldn't argue that. Being refused based on having special needs was something I was going to fight to the death! Strangely enough, before I even had time to sit down and write my appeal, quoting all the anti-discrimination legislation they were breaking, I received an after-hours call from the school principal's private mobile reluctantly saying the Department of Education had overruled his decision. Sebastian was now accepted back into the school. I was gob-smacked and utterly confused. My son was over the moon, shouting and jumping as he ran excitedly around the room. They asked for his subject selection (again), and on the last day of school, we had his timetable and group allocation. He was back in! A fight worth fighting, but surely the easier thing would have been for the school never to have changed their mind from their original offer months earlier. In the days before Christmas both my children had been accepted into the school and the kinder, we wanted after months of fighting, and I could finally breathe a sigh of relief.

WISDOM

I don't know it all, far from it in fact, and can't imagine what life is like for other families raising children on the spectrum. I do, however, think I've acquired a great deal from my parenting experiences that I would love to share. My biggest learning has been that parents know their children better than anyone, and we can trust our intuitions and be respected as the experts on our children. Always trust your gut. Secondly, we are the advocates for our children and the only ones who will keep on fighting for them. No matter how hard, or how much you are up against, we can never give up fighting for our kids to be the best version of themselves. To achieve this, they need to be able to access appropriate funding, services and education to truly shine. Finally, and probably most importantly, we need to love our children unconditionally. They are their own unique little selves, and while a diagnosis of ASD can help us understand their challenges, it can also remind us of their special talents, and they are lovable and perfect just as they are. Our children should never be changed to fit into a box, they will make their own distinctive mark on the world and make it a better place just by being part of it.

I bought a ticket for this rollercoaster when I chose to become a parent, and I'm riding over the bumps and challenges and speeding through the exhilarating joys on this ride of a lifetime two-fold. I wouldn't have it any other way.

CATHERINE ROSALION is one of Australia's leading Autism specialists. Through her business 'Autism Support' she has helped hundreds of families with children with Autism Spectrum Disorder (ASD) to lead happier and easier lives. She currently runs amazing sensory and social school holiday programs for children on the spectrum. Her passion for working with children with ASD blossomed from her experiences with her first therapy client when she was 17 years old. She studied a Bachelor of Behavioural Science (Psychology), completed a Diploma of Education and Master's in Special Education and has been dedicated to working in the field ever since! Catherine is also the proud single mother to two ausome children, Sebastian and Ava, who both have a diagnosis of ASD. As a teacher and a parent, Catherine has ridden the bumps of the ASD journey and understands the unsurmountable challenges and indescribable joys that can be found along this ride of a lifetime.

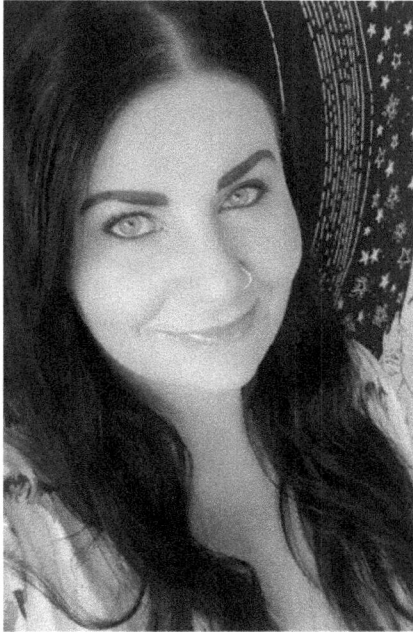

Big Love Revisited
by Anthea Flowers

DEC 30th, 2019

As I sit here and reflect on the past few years, I am amazed at the difference in our lives between when I last wrote for the *Parenting A Child on the Spectrum* book and now – chalk and cheese is an understatement!

When I last contributed, my son, who has Autism as well as comorbid ADHD and a tic disorder, was about to enter grade 4; he is now about to enter grade 8. My daughter is about to be in grade 9. Fully fledged teenagers with minds of their own, and no instruction manual! Although challenging, it has also allowed some of the best moments and experiences. Getting to see who our children are, and are evolving into, is indeed an honour.

So much has changed for me personally, in my career and definitely in my motherhood journey.

Just after I last wrote, my mother was diagnosed with stage IV inoperable pancreatic cancer. I was her primary carer as well as for the children, and I endured every sad, tragic and special moment along the way. Raising my son during this time was one of the hardest tasks I have ever been assigned; we did it, though. The experience bonded our trio even further. We were borne of the trauma, and the grief, through 11 months of heart wrenching care until her death. The funeral, and the aftermath, changed our lives forevermore.

My mum had worked at the Anglican school my children attended. Her sickness and then death was a massive upheaval in the everyday routine that my son had become so accustomed to. His once 'known' was obliterated. Everything seemed so different for him in the after. People treated him differently, no G'ma at school, constant reminders and of course big behaviours with not being able to process his emotions and all that change.

Our once well-oiled machine broke down, and none of the usual fixes did anything to restart it again.

We were back to square one.

I tried therapy for both of my children. Back to all of the specialists and searching for new strategies that could actually work or buy us some time. In this same timeframe, my ex-husband re-partnered and changed the dynamic of their once yearly visit with their dad from USA. My daughter was also diagnosed during this time with an anxiety disorder and skin picking disorder and they both severely impeded on her everyday life.

I had lost the only family I had where we lived. Now both my parents were deceased, and I was thrust into 'big sister aka fill-in mum' role for my older brother and two younger sisters as well. I had no support. One woman, feeling the weight of the world upon her. To be honest, it nearly crushed me. My own grief and loss at times was overwhelming, let alone trying to forge new ways for my son. But somehow, some way, one foot in front of the other, lots of error, and then some successes, it became easier in little ways.

It required a whole lot of me getting back to basics. Of giving my time, and of re-learning for myself what my son needed, required and what his new limits, likes and dislikes were. Then I had to feed this back through to the specialists, who only got an hour with him a week, and to his teachers, to try and provide them with strategies that would assist them with his in class and at school behaviours.

The school and teachers all looked to me as the 'all knowing' mother, wanting me to have all the answers, which as any of you with children with different modes of processing or needs know, is no easy feat! I was flying by the seat of my pants most of the time.

During this time, I also had to deal with the often-felt mistreatment and feelings from my daughter towards her brother, because after all, why was his behaviour fair, or why did she have to put up with a lot of his stuff? At home *and* at school. Why was I, as she saw, harder on her than her brother? Which no amount of explaining that being a parent to a kid on the spectrum means you are picking your battles seems fair to a sibling at that age!

I had to manage my time so efficiently so that I was there for my son in all of his moments, helping the school as much as possible, and to have special time with my daughter, plus trying to steal some mini moments for myself for self-care.

That would be the one constant between back then, and now, that self-care, and looking after myself well is paramount to the kind of mother I am. Lord knows I need the patience and ability to deal with the situations that can pop up out of nowhere, to take it all in stride, so self-care is the key to all of that. I notice when I suffer, when I am not doing what I need to for myself, not filling my own wellspring. That this is when my ship starts to sink, and of course my beauty-full son feeds off my own energy.

We came again to a place where we were coping, where we had some new strategies sorted out, communication with school was fairly good, and things were a bit easier.

Then, I re-partnered...

In hindsight I would not have made that choice; instead, it was a very big learning curve! I thought I had picked a decent partner, a police officer, older, he had kids at the same school, and I had waited 5yrs on my own before I started a relationship again. I think I was just lonely, I definitely settled, and that showed over the course of the relationship. My son (and daughter), both were not happy with the dynamic, with his kids, or the way our lives changed. For my son though, it was a loose thread that again unravelled all the hard work we had put in to get him to that previous coping spot.

In one swift swoop, we were right in the middle of a pretty bad relationship, with a very controlling man who did not in *any* way understand Autism or ADHD. His expectations of me, and of my son, were ridiculous. After 18 months the relationship ended very badly. It affected all three of us. We all had to start from scratch yet again – not only emotionally and financially, but also in our Autism journey.

Then came the hormones!

My son seemed to morph overnight into an angsty, angry, often violent, withdrawn mess. Teenage years are tricky to parent at the best of times – add in that extra dynamic of different sensory needs and processing, and it was an all-out shit show!

In light of the struggles my son was having at school with his new behaviours we actually looked to change his school, going from the private system and smaller classes to a larger public school that had more awareness and inclusivity to people on the spectrum and those with extra learning and behavioural needs. The change in schools has been both a blessing and a curse, allowing him space to just be – however, also teaching him some rather unsavoury vocabulary and other habits.

We started his year 7 year trying medication to assist with the distraction type behaviours to assist him in class time. It worked for a period, but the come down was horrendous. Every afternoon he would crash & burn and have an inevitable meltdown of epic proportions. He also ate rarely on the medication, and as a scrawny kid to begin with he really couldn't afford to lose more weight. Halfway through the year we stopped the medication, and while the in-class behaviours escalated, he was back to more manageable after school behaviours, normal weight and appetite.

In July 2019, I re-partnered again. This time, apart from teething problems in the first couple of months the relationship is very positive, and it has really helped my 12-year-old to have a good role model around, and someone who understands his ways of being. Having a man who can mentor and shape my son in the ways he needs has made his life more fruitful. My ex-husband and his wife had a baby in September 2019 which was a hard adjustment for my son as well, now having to share the little time yearly that he did have his dad with others. His non acceptance of that point is something we will work on – allowing the 'what is'.

It is a beautiful thing to see the moments where my son blooms, to see him confident in his skin. He has incorporated humour into his life to help him deal with his own Autism and ADHD, and often lightens the situation for himself, school, friends and family. That approach is not for everyone; however, it is empowering to him. No-one can ever bring him down because he happily takes the piss out of himself, a strategy that was not taught to him but rather something he discovered for himself as a coping mechanism.

We still have many hurdles ahead of us. There are many teenage years to still experience, but we are happy, whole, taking care of ourselves; and when things do happen, we approach it as a team: 'How can we deal with this or solve this?' And sometimes, it just is what it is, no solution necessary.

As a mother, I see we are still lacking in our education options for kids with Autism. The expectations placed on them to complete the normal curriculum and to conform is preposterous. In society, there is still much to be done to re-educate people about what having Autism actually means, or ADHD. The societal norms are what hinder and impede on your internal landscape. You have to give up the picture of the so-called 'normal' and make your peace with that. In letting go of the 'how it should be', we allow ourselves space to enjoy the 'what is'.

I'll be honest and say we did try the NDIS scheme, but we live in a regional coastal town, the options weren't great, and it was a lot of continued paperwork for something that didn't add to our lives, so we ditched the NDIS in favour of continuing to do things ourselves.

One other positive is that the public high school the kids now attend is very big on culture, and with our Wiradjuri Aboriginal heritage it has been such a blessing allowing my daughter to tap in dance, and having my son's language taught through school.

As my son grows, and as we go into 2020, there will be things that come up — challenges, roadblocks, behaviours, as well as successes, new friends, new interests and growth. I look forward to the gamut, because it has been through this parenting experience that I have become a better, more rounded, more understanding and empathetic person, mother and worker. Living with and raising someone with Autism and ADHD has expanded my world. I am no longer boxed in; I am open, I see different possibilities and perspectives. At the end of the day, my only advice is to take care of yourself, and to do what works for you. If it stops working, find something else that works. There is no perfect solution, no need to be anything, or do anything, other than what you are happy doing or being. That is what is important, that you know your child, work with them, help them to understand themselves, and ultimately, that you have connection and grow together throughout the journey. The rest is all just noise.

Whatever is good for your soul, do that; the same with your children. At the end of the day, to quote Ram Dass, 'we are all just walking each other home.'

ANTHEA FLOWERS is a mum of two teenagers, step mum to three bonus teenagers, one primary schooler and three adults!

Anthea is a social worker, youth worker and counsellor. She is also a mentor and works in a community centre. Her passion is our youth, connecting with them and helping them with where they are at.

Anthea is also involved in The Red Dust Healing program, which comes from an Indigenous perspective on healing.

In her busy life, she advocates for kids, youth and teens, particularly those who do not fit into the schooling system and have different abilities and needs.

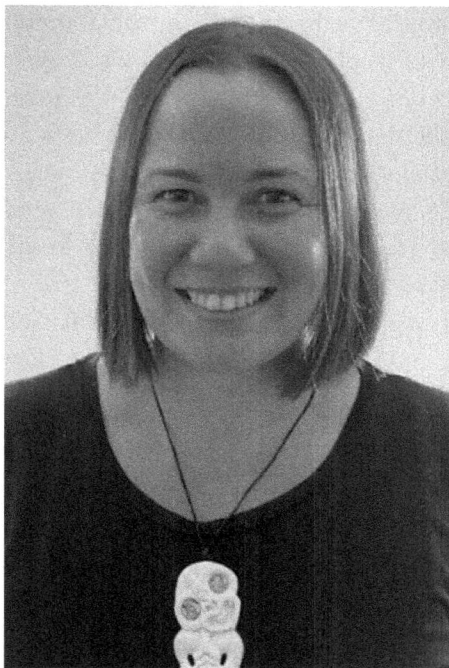

Becoming Jaden
by Leah Adam

It's been quite the journey for us!

The world in which we live is a confusing and strange place where human beings are forced into boxes and labelled. We don't all fit a box or a label, and that is OK.

CJ was really struggling in this world. CJ didn't fit in and self-harming was fast becoming a very dangerous and almost daily habit. High school was awful, and the constraints on CJ to conform to be 'normal' to behave in an appropriate way was absolute torture!

There was a video clip doing the rounds on social media of an iguana being chased by snakes and CJ saw this and said that was how it felt every single day when she went to school. I was horrified that I was putting my child through this humiliation and torture every day. Most days were awful, and it got to the point where I was receiving phone calls daily, sometimes even multiple – mostly the same stuff, e.g. CJ refused to follow instructions, refused work, refused to co-operate in a group assignment, refused to go to sport etc. etc. etc. At one point there was a standoff with a teacher and the rest of the class was evacuated ... it was just a power struggle war and it didn't end well. It was a traumatic experience and CJ never returned to that school.

We found an alternative school, and in 12 months CJ had achieved a Certificate 2 in animal studies, participated in activities, made friends and got along with the teacher – somewhat! We still had good and bad days, and sometimes CJ was just too exhausted to attend, it was just so draining physically and mentally – she really only coped with 3 days of school, even with the short 4-hour school days.

One day, CJ confided in me that she was not a girl but a boy. This was not the first time CJ had said this and my initial response was 'no, you are a girl, don't be silly.' CJ has always been a tomboy and I honestly just thought she was gay and just brushed it off ... for a number of years. When this came up again, I talked about teenage hormones and how we are all different and get confused but all I got was, 'No, mum, I think I am a transgender male.' I had no real idea about transgender stuff. We spoke with our psychologist about it and we were referred to the gender clinic.

My main concern was how would she know at such a young age? What if she changed her mind? How could we be sure this wasn't just a phase, mixed in with ASD and anxiety and not quite fitting in and all – I was totally and utterly confused. The gender clinic people were fantastic and put it all in black and white for us and I finally understood ... in a nutshell, my child was trapped in the wrong body so at every turn looking in the mirror, showering, wearing dresses, growing breasts, this was all so traumatic for CJ ... the clinic recommended social transitioning, where you transition socially just changing your name and pronouns. We didn't even know what that meant. But it had really became a life or death situation and having our child in so much pain tore us all apart.

I was overloaded with questions... How would I tell my family? What would they say? What about my grandparents, would they understand? Would our family still love us? Would they disown us? Will my child be picked on and ridiculed? This is not a life someone just *chooses* to live ... so many thoughts rushing through my mind! You read so much negative stuff that you just can't help but be drawn there. My husband Dan is an amazing man; he is a practical man, a carpenter, a bloke's bloke. He wears singlets and thongs, drinks stubbies, and is the eldest of 5 boys (no sisters) – and he was just like, 'Yep, ok, we got this.' I am so lucky to have him as our glue as I was just quietly falling apart! This was certainly not the path I ever thought we would be on. He puts everything into perspective, and just like that we tell some of our close family and friends. Most were unphased and just ran with it, some questions arose but after a few educational conversations most understood and supported us. If they didn't like it – too bad. People always say that I'm strong, and I do try to be, but Dan is a pillar of strength for me. We are so lucky to have such amazing support. I didn't start attending pride marches or screaming from the roof tops that my child is transgender or anything crazy like that, but I love my child unconditionally and this is just another experience for us all we are all in this together as family. Many friends and extended family members weren't told immediately, but over time those conversations will be had as required. You don't just pick up the phone and start ringing distant relatives to say 'Hey, my child is trans.'

So, just like that, our CJ became our Jaden.

(From here on in, Jaden will be referred to using the correct pronouns.)

The school was a relatively new school, and Jaden was the first trans person to attend. The transitioning at school wasn't successful, and they were not as supportive as we had hoped. Initially they asked us if we would like to move campuses, as there was another trans student at the other Brisbane campus. Students were great, but the staff not so much. One teacher would purposely use Jaden's old name and pretty much refused to use the correct pronouns, which usually created an argument. Then I would get the phone call to come and collect Jaden from school. This eventually became a huge problem, and Jaden started refusing school again, eventually finishing year 10 and not returning. I have had to quit numerous jobs due to Jaden being unpredictable and requiring full time support. This has been a really difficult for us all, both mentally and financially.

At home, things have improved greatly. Jaden was really happy with his new name and seemed to be coping really well. I was shocked at how much this name change had improved his confidence. We have since changed Jaden's name on all legal documents, and this process was at times really hard... the lady at Medicare was asking why we changed his name, and was clearly not supportive; she didn't even process the paperwork, which resulted in another trip to the Medicare office to start the whole process again 3 months later. So, every appointment we attended would result in the doctor's office calling out Jaden's old name, which caused many a meltdown. Now that we have the official name change, appointments are far less stressful. Recently, at a clinic appointment for Jaden's ultrasound, the practice manager called me in to their office privately, which immediately made my heart race, thinking the worst and that medically something was terribly wrong. She had called me in to ask for my advice as they wanted to update their paperwork but didn't want to offend anyone, so I helped them decide how best to be able to be inclusive on the forms and still provide the necessary information. For example, you can't tick male on the forms when you are going in for an ultrasound of your ovaries and not expect the receptionist to be totally and utterly confused! You can, however, tick male and have a separate box for sex at birth, hence giving some clarity to the staff. I have since been back to this clinic where the updated forms were easy to fill out and certainly give us some peace of mind.

Health wise, Jaden has had a pretty rough time. He has been diagnosed with Polycystic Ovary Syndrome, which makes it tough when going to see gynaecologists when you are a man; it is pretty tricky and can often be confusing for all involved. We have been lucky finding a specialist who made us all feel comfortable. Jaden also struggles daily with chronic pain throughout his body, and we are currently looking at a possible diagnosis of fibromyalgia. His mental health is still up and down, and we have some good days and some very bad days.

The past year has included many positive improvements for Jaden. He has researched for quite some time the benefits of animal assistance, and to his credit has designed and planned a training schedule as well as identified the best animal for his needs. We are very proud of Jaden for taking the initiative to gather all this information. This year we have purchased a puppy as a companion for Jaden. We are hoping to train this puppy to be an assistance dog. This would greatly help him and his anxiety in the community as well as giving him some purpose and reason to leave the house and do some physical exercise. This hasn't all been smooth and according to schedule; as per usual there has been a few bumps along the way. To his credit, he has accepted that things will not always go to plan and he has remained focused in his task to train his new puppy. We have also engaged a professional for training and assistance which will commence shortly.

Today, Jaden is 16. We are only just starting the journey of getting support through the NDIS. We have gained access and are eagerly waiting our first planning meeting. We constantly worry about the future for Jaden, and we are trying to find some kind of balance in our lives. It is hard. For our family, life is chaotic and sometimes it's a whole lot of crazy, but we just do our best every day with the unconditional love and support of our big crazy family and some pretty special friends.

LEAH ADAM *is a 40-year-old fun loving mum of three amazing children: Tahliah (20), Jaden (17) and Lillian (14). She and her husband Dan are very lucky to have a large supportive network of family and friends.*

Having an Autistic transgender child certainly has its challenges.

Leah works part time at Autism Qld as a teacher's aide, a role that has given her the opportunity to work with families who inspire her. Leah hopes that by sharing her family's story others will gain comfort in knowing they are not alone.

Becoming Jaden
by Leah Adam

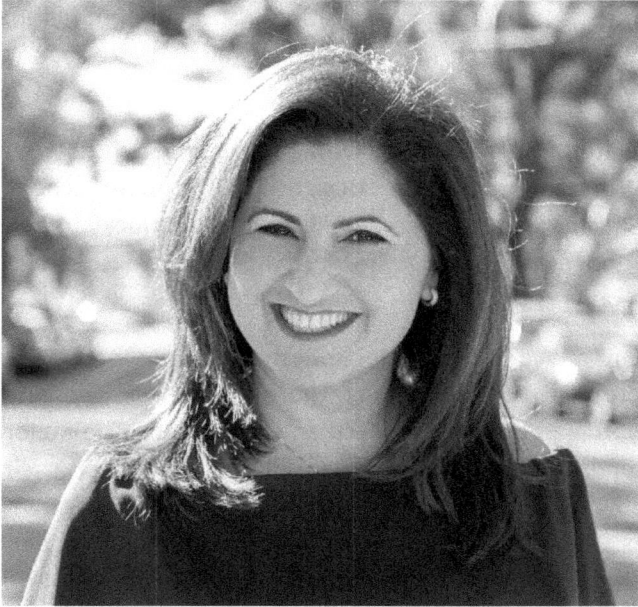

It's All About MATES!
by Randa Habelrih

Wow, wow, wow…. So much has happened since our last instalment of this amazing compilation! Richard had just completed high school and was looking to find his place in the world, and I had launched my book *Dealing with Autism* and thought that would be it regarding my role in advocacy!

If I had that crystal ball that I often refer to, and if I could have looked into the future, there is no way I could have imagined what our lives would look like.

I am in awe of the young man Richard has become and I am motivated to continue to agitate for change for all our young people on the Autism spectrum.

It has by no means been an easy transition from school to life in the big wide world; we have experienced many challenges along the way, and continue to do so, but the future looks bright!

Richard completed his transition to work programme, which was a post school government funded programme designed to prepare school leavers for employment. Richard learned many skills and he was lucky to be in the care of a dedicated and professional team, but did this lead to a successful work outcome? No.

He did do a stint at a local tennis club, but that did not work out. We were once again, forced to think outside the box. There are not many employers willing or able to give young people like Richard an opportunity. The major department stores and supermarkets informed us that they had filled their quotas and usually those who were lucky enough to be employed, held on tightly to these rare positions. These employees were loyal, reliable and eager to work. One would think that employers would recruit more, but that is not the case.

Richard and I sat down one day, and I asked him what he wanted to do.

He did not hesitate in his reply.

He stated, 'Mum, I like to work with children. I like to have fun and talk.'

Then he said, 'I really liked it when I spoke at your book launch and I told everyone that I am just like everyone else. I liked talking on the microphone.'

The penny dropped.

Richard is a natural public speaker. He has no fear of the stage, no fear of getting up in front of an audience and speaking, in fact he LOVES it. This is in stark contrast to studies which have found that people's number one fear is public speaking. Followed by death at number 2!

Even Jerry Seinfeld finds this intriguing. He puts this statistic into perspective... **'That means, to the average person, if you have to go to a funeral, you're better off in the casket than doing the eulogy.'**

At the same time that my book, *Dealing with Autism,* and the subsequent chapter in *Parenting A Child on the Spectrum* were launched, I was very much focused on developing the MATES Programme, an anti-bullying and social inclusion program for school students. No matter where someone is on the Autism spectrum, socialisation is often a huge challenge.

We all crave friendship; we all need a MATE. Our values are underpinned by the concept of MATESHIP; it's is a part of our Australian DNA. The reality is that no matter how wonderful our teachers are, they can't replicate the friendship from peers which children seek, and exclusion is very often the first form of bullying.

The MATES focus is on educating the entire student cohort on the subject of Autism and empowering a group of students with leadership skills.

What is MATES?

1. MATES is an acronym for **M**ates **A**ssisting **T**o **E**ngage **S**ocially
2. It's a simple concept; a proactive rather than a reactive solution to exclusion.
3. School MATES is a school-based, peer-led social inclusion *and* leadership program.
4. School MATES pairs students: one plays a leadership role by socially supporting a peer who may have difficulty with socialisation.
5. The MATES leader is recognized as part of the school leadership team – creating more leadership opportunities for students.

Outcomes for Students	**Outcomes for Schools**
o Creates a sense of belonging at school for all students	o Creates a more caring and engaged student cohort
o Empowers students to believe they can make a difference	o Social Justice is concretely implemented at school
o Develops a sense of empathy	o Creates a paradigm shift in school culture by empowering students to lead the change and reset the standards of inclusion
o Leadership skills are nurtured	
o High peer expectations of fellow students are established	o Moves the onus from teachers to students
o Allows students to challenge the status quo	o Can reduce negative behaviour in class triggered by frustration
	o Students' sense of belonging promotes a more settled class

Online support group for parents and families

At the same time, I established an online Facebook support group called Autism MATES primarily for parents because I recall how isolated I felt as a mother, and recall how I would have loved to be in contact with others who were experiencing similar challenges with their children.

The purpose of the group is to provide an engaged community where parents, siblings and teachers of young people on the Autism spectrum can connect.

In this group, the focus is on positivity and inspiration, and inclusion is our mantra. It's a group where members are encouraged to:

• Engage, collaborate and learn from each other

- Focus on the positives, and know that a different world is not the end of the world
- Share experiences and make a positive difference to the lives of those living with Autism
- Be a part of a movement that will change attitudes and raise the standards of inclusion

Together as a group, we will support each other as parents and carers, as well as strive to give our young people a voice and help create a more inclusive community. Autism MATES is not just a support group, it is an active group with a mission.

Events that empower young people on the spectrum

Autism MATES is all about empowerment. The support group empowers parents and carers, but we also run events to empower those on the spectrum. Our events are not presented from a pity platform or sense of victimhood. We run 2 key events which celebrate and empower our young people on the spectrum.

- The first of our events is Model MATES.

This is an annual modelling event where our models rock the catwalk alongside professional models to showcase the season's latest looks. This event is a metaphor highlighting that even in the most elite of industries, our young people on the spectrum can be included and rise to the occasion when given the opportunity. We hold our event in the elite arena of fashion and modelling, where they walk alongside professional models. We do not use a school hall but have the event hosted at a premiere shopping mall.

You may ask how would this be empowering?

Firstly, we style each model individually with the expert guidance of our stylist extraordinaire: Bernadette Payne of *That's My Style*. The models are consulted, and their input is valuable in creating their 'on trend' look. They interact with our stylist and learn to own their chosen look.

The effect on our models cannot be underestimated. It is POWERFUL to watch. They rise to the occasion; they are styled, and they feel invincible. It's truly amazing what some positive reinforcement can do!

Too often the focus is on their deficits and what they can't do. This event is about encouraging them to stand tall, hold their heads high and shine. They are fussed over by hairdressers, makeup artists, stylists and photographers; made to feel and look their absolute best... then they confidently strut their stuff on the catwalk in front of a cheering crowd!

The power of this positivity can change the trajectory of a young person's life. It takes courage and determination, but they have it, and they light up the catwalk. The skills and confidence which they learn from this experience are transformative.

This is what happens when you give our young people a platform to shine!

The Model MATES Event is about shifting the perspective of the way society views our young people. It's about celebrating their achievements and allowing them to express themselves.

But this event is not just about showcasing the season's latest trends and empowering our models, it's also about sending a message to the community that our young people on the Autism spectrum need to be recognised, included and made to feel that they contribute.

Whether it is inclusion in schools and the need for friendship, or the need to feel valued by having employment, we all have a personal role to play in creating a more inclusive society.

Each one of us can personally contribute... How, you may ask?

1. Try extending the hand of friendship to those who find social interaction challenging.
2. If you are in a position to do so, employ our young people. 1 in 5 Australians have a disability, and 65% of people on the Autism spectrum are unemployed. If you employ our young people, you are tapping into a new target market because these young people have parents and siblings and we will be loyal to you and your brand! Corporations and businesses spend their marketing budgets seeking new customers... well... here is an untapped market on a silver platter! So, in this increasingly competitive market, businesses should embrace our buying power!

I would like to invite other Westfield Centres and shopping malls to host Model MATES events so that this simple message can be spread far and wide.

I thank Westfield Eastgardens for their trail blazing and genuine efforts in corporate social responsibility. Too often we see big business merely paying lip service to the importance of their 'ties to the community' and their sense of social justice. This is social justice in *action*.

Model MATES is not a charity or fundraising event – it's an event which raises the profile of our children and creates a ripple of change for acceptance in our wider community. We present our children in a positive light and provide an alternative to counter the well-meaning advocates who pull out the pity card. Our children are to be celebrated, not pitied. They need opportunity, not charity. That is the Model MATES message. Model MATES is a call for inclusion.

- Our second event is The Autism MATES Speakers Conference.

This event is about giving our young people on the Autism spectrum the stage and the opportunity to advocate for themselves using their own voice. It's an opportunity to listen to our young people as they share with us their hopes and dreams. It's a chance for our community to have a glimpse into their lives, to be inspired by how they overcome challenges daily, and to come together to celebrate their achievements.

The event's goals:

1. The main goal is to present to our community, the humanity behind an Autism diagnosis and the different faces of the spectrum.
2. Another goal is to disrupt the current model of 'Autism conferences' whereby international experts and researchers are flown in at great expense to speak about those on the spectrum. These speakers traditionally have little experience other than that in a clinical setting. These experts are usually given top billing while those on the spectrum are given token billing on a side stage and are expected to volunteer their time and to also pay the exorbitant entry fee.
3. It is my goal to hold an Autism MATES speaking event in every state and to make it a major focus, not only on the Autism calendar but also on the education calendar.

At the Autism MATES events, our speakers on the spectrum are respected and paid for their time and expertise. This event is about giving our young people on the spectrum a platform and a voice.

It is time they are given the opportunity to advocate for themselves; enough of other people speaking for them and on their behalf. **Just because they may have difficulty speaking, does not mean they have nothing to say.**

Somewhere along this journey, my child became the teacher.

I have learned more about life from my son than from anything or anyone else in this world. I celebrate my son and his peers. They overcome daily obstacles that most people would not encounter in a lifetime. These young, tenacious people have a story, which is worth sharing.

Public speaking is challenging enough for most people but when you add communication challenges to the mix, it is even more daunting. Congratulations to all our speakers who stand up on that stage and refuse to use their Autism diagnosis as an excuse!

If you ever have the opportunity to attend this event, make sure you come along. If you would like this event hosted in your city, get in touch, it is a regular event in Sydney and we have held an event in Brisbane, it's now your city's turn.

Join us in breaking down barriers and be a part of the solution!

Best MATES puppet show

The Best MATES puppet show is the brainchild of my son Richard and is based on his experiences of bullying and exclusion in schools. He presents this to primary schools students.

The puppet show brings the MATES message to primary school and pre-school students in a fun and interactive way. We believe that if you want to change the world, the best place to start is with our children!

The Best MATES Puppet Show is a story about the friendship between Tommy the Turtle and Danny the Duck. We feel that it's time to take the negativity out of the subject of bullying and inject some fun and storytelling into this very serious and real problem; a problem that is becoming more prevalent and damaging to so many of our young people.

Tommy the Turtle doesn't really fit in the ocean or the land; Richard plays the role of Tommy, and in doing so, Richard gives Tommy an authentic voice, as he himself was subjected to extreme bullying all through school because he did not quite 'fit in' due to his Autism.

This is not a story about Autism – it's a story of difference, and just like Richard, Tommy did not quite fit in.

Richard first shares his own school journey with school students in his speech, 'I'm Just Like Everyone Else'. A speech he has told many times over and has impacted thousands of students. Following this, Richard brings Tommy to life as students to sit back and enjoy the adventures of Tommy & Danny.

The goal of Best MATES is to promote inclusion and try to prevent bullying from occurring, instead of trying to address the issue once it has manifested.

We would love to take Tommy and Danny to every primary school in the country, which is why we are now exploring the possibility of creating a cartoon animation of the puppet show. This way the MATES message can reach even the most remote rural school in the country, and who knows, maybe Tommy will become known internationally!

For the past 4 years I had been working hard putting these events on. During this time, they had all been self-funded. It was time to scale our efforts in order to scale our impact, so we started the process of registering Autism MATES as a charity. We were thrilled to achieve this status as this now allows us the opportunity to apply for grants and to fundraise so that we can take these events all over the country.

The grant writing space is new to me and is a challenging one, but I am determined to crack the code. I am also in the process of trying to recruit volunteers, as the dream grows bigger each day and I need help in making the dreams a reality for our children, who deserve the same opportunities as everyone else.

The MATES Café

My aim is to now scale the success and events of the past 5 years so that we can reach more people. Now that Autism MATES is a registered charity, I am working towards the next goal, The MATES Café.

The inspiration of course is Richard, my amazing, engaging, funny, 23-year-old son who, despite his unique skills and genuine desire to work, is still looking to find his place in our world. Employers are not rolling out the red carpet for him and he hates not having a sense of worth. He is not alone.

According to the ABS, 'the labour force participation rate is 40.8% among the 75,200 people of working age (15-64 years) living with Autism spectrum disorders.'

There are few options for school leavers who are on the Autism spectrum other than adult babysitting services that suck NDIS funding and provide no outcomes. Unfortunately, we have little choice but to send him to one of these services because Richard hates waking up and having no plan for the day. So, we access the best service we can find, but it's not good enough.

Richard has a capacity to learn and contribute, and so do many of his peers.

We have created opportunities for him. He speaks at schools and conferences and performs his puppet show to preschools and primary schools all over Australia. This is an amazing outcome for a child who was non-verbal, and one whom many expected would not graduate from high school.

While he very much enjoys these opportunities that provide him with an income, albeit an inconsistent one, Richard craves routine. He also craves socialisation and wants to learn and engage with the community.

The MATES Café will provide the opportunity to teach our young people hospitality skills, and for those who can take these skills out to open employment that will be a huge win. For those who will need to stay in this supported environment, they will have a social enterprise that will employ and teach them skills as opposed to 'babysitting' them. This model is not one based on segregation, as it requires the support of the local community to buy their coffee/lunch, have meetings and catch-ups, and place boardroom catering orders from this café. Patrons will interact with our young people and help them feel that they belong to our community. An important goal is also for the café to be profitable, so that the model can be replicated.

Our young people do not want charity or welfare, they want genuine opportunity.

I would like to emphasise that Autism MATES is not about garnering pity, it is about embracing the idea of helping our young people become economically independent. It's not about 'giving them a fish', it's about 'teaching them to fish'.

Our society is too entrenched in a welfare mentality, and that's not what our young people want; they want opportunity. Our goal is to work towards shifting the over-reliance on handouts and segregated day-programmes for our young people with Autism.

MATES Awards

Since the MATES awards is all about empowerment, it was only natural that we created our Autism MATES Awards. Our inaugural awards were launched at our first Christmas fundraising lunch and we were thrilled to honour the beacons of light in industry, schools and community, who make such a huge difference to our young people on the Autism spectrum.

We had 6 categories, these included:

The Corporate MATES Award

For exemplary Corporate Social Responsibility and inclusive practice for the Autism community.

- Westfield Eastgardens

The Business MATES Award

For small businesses or entrepreneurs who have displayed leadership and implemented inclusive practices.

- That's My Style by Bernadette

The School MATES Award

For a mainstream school that has implemented programmes or practices which encourage inclusion of students on the spectrum.

- Moriah College

The Little MATES Award

For Early Educators who demonstrate leadership and inclusive practice for our little ones on the spectrum.

- Michelle Bouabaid
- All Star Learners

The Best MATES Peer Award

For an organisation that works specifically and collaboratively for inclusion and support for the Autism community.

- Autism Community Network

The Shooting Star Award

For an individual on the Autism spectrum who has overcome challenges and made a significant impact in serving to inspire his peers.

-    Richard Habelrih

I have invited each of our winners to be on the judging panel for this year's awards. There will be a nomination process and entries will be invited from all over the country. We want to acknowledge those who are doing good. This follows our mantra of empowerment and positivity.

What's working out there and what's not?

The biggest challenge that we are facing is that there is so much that needs to be done. Our organisation is volunteer based, but it is now time to grow. I am frustrated by the huge amounts of funds that are being allocated to the same groups of people. The funding exists but it is challenging to break into the tight circle. As a society, we need to think more innovatively, because our children deserve a better outcome than is currently on offer.

What are we working toward now? Where do we want to be in the next 4 years?

If I had that crystal ball and I could look into the future, I would love to see:

1. The MATES café successfully and profitably operating, and employing our community;
2. The Best MATES Puppet Show animation a reality and being distributed to all primary schools;
3. School MATES in all high schools;

4. Model MATES featured in Sydney Fashion week, as well as interstate; and
5. Autism MATES Speakers Conference held in cities outside of Sydney.

Because at the end of the day, it's all about MATES – it's all about feeling that we belong.

RANDA HABELRIH is the founder and director of Autism MATES, a registered charity and social enterprise, with a vision to empower those living on the autism spectrum. Randa is a passionate advocate and voice for those on the spectrum and their families, an award-winning speaker, author, and mother of an amazing young man with autism.

Her work has been recognised internationally, having won Gold in the 'Women Helping Women' category and Silver for 'Best New Product or Service' for MATES in the 2017 International Women in Business Stevie Awards. She also received a Women's Economic Forum award in 2019. Randa is passionate about changing the standards of social inclusion of our young people on the spectrum, but she is most proud of the fact that her son, who she was told would never talk, is now advocating for himself and his peers, and is a sought-after keynote speaker.

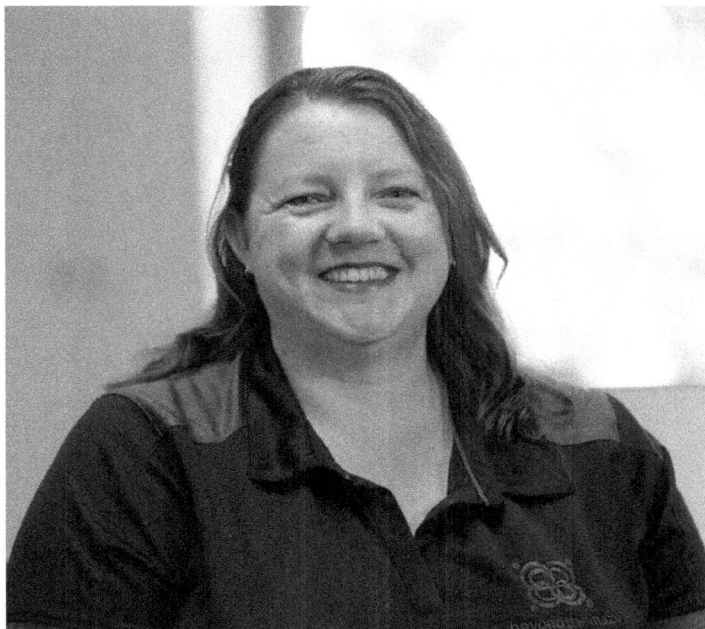

The School That Changed Everything!
by Paula Burgess

How so much can change in a few years! In my last chapter I had left you with our story of JB being expelled from day-care and considering home-schooling after what it seemed that every option we thought about didn't want to help us, and feeling like everything was just falling down around us. We had a lot of school challenges with the feeling that he didn't quite fit into the schooling system, but we just didn't know what to do about it.

I had given up my full-time employment as a financial planner and started my own business so I could be around to support JB through his schooling, and this was definitely the right choice for us given the support he needed.

We had followed the Failsafe diet and found some great results from using that, but it certainly didn't 'fix' anything, and we were being pressured to medicate as the school was struggling to 'handle' him.

We got a dog to help him regulate this feelings and was going to train him to be his assistance dog, however that never came to reality as the dog ended up being too anxious and obsessed over JB to be able to be trained as an assistance dog. If I had to guess, I would say that the dog also has ADHD, and when the two of them escalate it is bedlam in this house!

We were about to head into Year 2 at the time of all of that being written, and it seems so very long ago, with some definite highs and lows along the way.

Now we are about to head into Year 6, and it has certainly been an interesting ride.

After we looked at different schools throughout Prep and Year 1 and found that no one really wanted to take him, we stayed with where we were. This wasn't a bad school at all, in fact I really liked it; it was just that he didn't fit the mould of the school system, and this is where we all struggled. Like all schools, you have a mix of teachers, and some work better than others.

My last resort was an all-boys school about 30 – 40 minutes' drive from us that may have been the answer, but that didn't start until Year 5, so I put his name down there and continued at the school we had.

Over the years at school, I spent my time continually working with the teachers and advocating for my son. I kept asking for him to be challenged at school, given that he was so academically switched on, but unfortunately the behaviour continued to overshadow the need to challenge him academically.

I took matters into my own hands when it came to academics and purchased those academic books that you get from the newsagent. I purchased the ones that were a year or two above his year level at school, and he loved them.

In the meantime, I started to look closer into the all-boys school that I had put his name down for. I went to a couple of their open days and just loved everything that they stood for. I finally thought I had found somewhere that JB was going to fit into and thrive in. We got an interview, and I was so excited! As scared as I was about being honest with them, I knew that I have to be as I didn't want him going into the school under false pre-tenses, they had to know what they were agreeing to. We had the interview, and I think JB talked the lady's ear off, but she seemed quite taken with him.

Surprisingly to me, JB wanted to go to this school and I wanted him to go there, but I had my reservations about moving him. At his current school he spent most of his time socialising with the girls, and yet I was ready to throw him into a school with only boys! I was worried, but deep down I just knew somehow that this was going to be the right move for him.

However, the universe seemed to have other ideas, and we didn't get accepted. Deep down I was devasted as I really thought this would work for him, however I had been here before, it was just another step in our journey. Although, something was also niggling at me telling me that he would be accepted and to just be patient.

We moved into year 4 at our existing school and we got a fantastic teacher who was not only tough but saw his ability and strong desire to do the harder work. Although, in many of my meetings with her, she did mention that he was one of the more challenging students she has ever had in her teaching career (and she was about to retire!), but she never gave up on him. She could see that he was destined for great things and didn't want to squash that.

She was certainly tough on him when she needed to be, and JB struggled with this, but once he saw that his father and I had her back and agreed with everything she was doing for him, he was resigned to the fact that he wasn't going to win those battles.

We had reached a point where although he was still unmedicated we didn't need our therapists any longer. We had changed our psychologist yet again and found someone amazing, and after seeing her for a while, we felt we could do it without her and come back if needed. She ended up working with me in the conferences I had been running and other courses we were writing, so she was confident I knew what I was doing.

Part way through Year 4, I was sitting at my desk working away at my computer and I saw an email pop up from the school I wanted JB to go to. An opening had been made available and they had accepted him at the school. I think I screamed and cried at the same time. I knew this feeling was right, he was going to this school. I really hoped this was the right move for him.

We had put so much work into his current school and we were on such a nice communication level with them by now that things were moving along nicely. To move him from something that was working OK to a totally new environment was so scary!

I braced myself to tell him that he was going to this school (I hadn't told him that he didn't get accepted the first time as my gut told him that he would be, so I didn't need to bother him). I sat him down and said, 'Do you remember that school we went to a couple of times that you really liked?' He said yes. 'Well, you have been accepted, and you will be going next year.'

He jumped off his chair and did a happy dance. Well, I didn't need to be worried about that then, did I?

Over the course of the year, we did many things to help with the transition. We spoke about who he wasn't going to see anymore, how the new school would work, we took a few drives over to where the school was … the school themselves did some absolutely awesome transition appointments, even though my car wheel was damaged on the way to one of them (which was a group one with other kids unfortunately) resulting in us missing an appointment.

The School That Changed Everything!
by Paula Burgess

He handled the entire process so well, and the school was awesome about booking another appointment.

The day finally came where we did our final orientation and took him to meet his 'big brother'. The school has a 'big brother' program where the Year 5 boys are matched with a Year 12 boy to help them through their first year at the new school. We were so fortunate to be matched with the school captain, though I didn't realise how lucky we really were until later in that first school year. This big brother was amazing, and what a role model for JB!

We started Year 5 with apprehension. I was so worried about how he was going to go in a new school and whether this was the right move for him, but he started the day with excitement!

The school requested that we leave the boys at the school gate, and their big brothers would come and meet them. Wow! This was hard! After years of me having to take him to his classroom as the year always started with apprehension and the real possibility of a meltdown, this year I had to leave him to his own feelings and allow him to process them by himself. Our first experience of this school treating the boys as young men and helping them move into manhood.

With tears in my eyes and my heart pounding so hard in my chest that I thought I might jump out of there, I gave him a kiss and hug goodbye for the day and off he went, with a packed school back so big that it was half his size! His big brother was walking down the driveway with a big smile on his face and a wave to tell us 'We've got this', and off they went.

I spend the entire day worrying how he was going, but of course, I didn't need to!

I picked him up at the end of the day and he was so full of energy, bursting to tell me all about his first day and the new school war cry that he had learned.

This enthusiasm continued throughout the year! I never once had a problem getting him out the door to go to school – he was itching to get there! He immersed himself in school activities, both in and out of school times, joined a soccer and swim team, and loved it! He had never been into sports before and honestly, he isn't particularly great at sports, but he gave it a go. There were so many other kids that were obviously part of swimming and soccer clubs outside of school and were so much better than him, but he didn't care; he was loving it, so he just kept going.

The school saw how he was excelling academically within the first term and invited him to be part of an honours program that they run for kids who are excelling, so you could imagine my excitement! Finally, someone seeing his true potential! He loved that, too!

I could see a boy that had struggled through school the past 5 years, finally being able to spread his wings and fly!

He had a wonderful male teacher as well, and this was the first time that he had a male teacher throughout his entire years at school and day-care. I think this was one of the best teachers to start with. Being at an all-boys school, the majority of the teachers are male, which I think is going to be the best thing for JB over the coming years.

JB loves performing arts. He may not excel in sport, but he does the arts! He was able to be part of the choir and a music program and is trying out for the school musical next year.

The school knows what I do with my coaching and are very open to my feedback but honestly, I haven't needed to give them any. I am so confident that they know what they are doing, they have got this.

I remember going to my first IEP meeting with the school and sitting down, listening to the learning support teacher and JB's teacher and thinking, 'they are all over his needs.' Not to mention the fact that ADHD doesn't come with any funding in school, so they didn't have to do IEP's for him, but they did them anyway! After discussing his plan, they handed it over to me and said, 'you have a look over it and tell us if there is anything we are missing or that you need done.' I had a look and said, 'No, you guys have got this completely, there is nothing I would add to that at all!'

Now, I won't say that this has been a totally seamless process for us at all. It has had its ups and downs, although not many. Firstly, he was the only boy that had come over from his school, so it took a while for him to find 'his people', which led to a few issues with bullying and other kids giving him a bit of a hard time. However, the policy his school has around bullying and how it is handled is fantastic in itself, so it was quickly nipped in the bud, so to speak.

As it can take 40 minutes to get to the school in peak hour traffic, it also takes a lot more of my own time to get him to and from school, but he did express an interest in catching the bus which meant I only need to drive him 10 minutes up the road to get it. However, it was a scary move and I wasn't sure he was ready for it. Term 3 rolled around, and we discussed it again. His big brother also caught the same bus, so we organised for me to drive him to the same stop his big brother caught the bus at so they could go together. I was OK with this. He loved it! He wanted to do it a lot more, but we decided to ease him into it. By the end of Term 4, he was catching the bus almost every day! It was certainly something I didn't see him doing for some time, so it was a huge step for us. Although it did help immensely that this bus was only for his school, so there were no bus changes at all.

I can honestly say that with one year of this new school behind us that it has certainly changed all our lives in a positive way, and we look forward to our coming years as part of this school.

As what happens with many ADHD children, puberty has hit early, so we are now faced with other challenges that, honestly, I don't think I am quite ready for.

We have gone back to our psychologist recently as there are a few things in JB's life that he seems to be struggling with; pre-teen attitude and stubbornness is hitting hard and is definitely putting my training and strategies to the test, and the thoughts of medication are back on the table as well.

JB has been learning to meditate as well, which is a huge part of my life, and I believe that I can help him to work through his feelings and reactions with things if meditation is part of his. The most important thing I have heard him take on from my teachings is that he cannot control anyone else's actions and feelings, only his own, and that has helped him work through things incredibly.

Going forward, I believe that there will always be challenges and struggles with some parts of our life, but we just need to think about what they are teaching us and how to get through them. I see the school being such a positive influence in his life for some time and will help to form the wonderful man he will become.

My tips for you going forward are:

LISTEN TO YOUR GUT – Your gut is rarely wrong! If it is telling you that it is the right thing to do, no matter how scary, then it probably is. When I decided on this school and we were accepted, I was so scared about how JB would handle the move, but deep down my instincts were telling me that it was definitely the right move so I stuck with it and they were right! Really get in tune with what your gut is telling you and run with it!

MEDITATE – I can honestly say that meditation has changed my life! Meditating every day has helped me deal with even the most stressful of things and remain calm in the time of need. I am now teaching JB the value of meditation, and quite often I will head to my bedroom to do an hour-long meditation and JB will join me. So many people say that you can't teach anyone with ADHD how to meditate as they can't keep still, but I can honestly tell you that you can, it takes a little longer but you certainly can reap the benefits.

YOU CAN ONLY CONTROL YOURSELF! – The most valuable thing I have taught JB is that you can't control what others say or do, just how you react to it. I have also taught him that if someone is saying or doing something mean to you, it generally means that this is a reflection of something in themselves that they don't like. Now, to an 11-year-old this is a hard concept to grasp, but I know that as I have been teaching him this for about 2 – 3 years now it has helped him through so many things!

To those just starting their journeys I can honestly say that things will get better. As hard as it feels things get sometimes, just try and find the positive in things and focus on that! It *will* get better.

PAULA BURGESS *is a mum of a wonderful young boy diagnosed with ADHD who changed her career path in a way she never imagined. Paula now works with parents and children affected by ADHD. She sees children with ADHD as 'world changers' and works with them to help them to be the best people they can be.*

Paula believes that if we teach people how to understand and accept ADHD then it will not only open more opportunities, but it will give them permission to fly.

Paula has coached, supported and advocated for many parents of children with ADHD and worked with some wonderful children. She has given many talks to various childcare centres and conferences to educate parents on what support is available and provided educators with ideas to provide a supported classroom. She has been interviewed by various media outlets spreading the word about ADHD.

Paula is an ADDCA trained ADHD Coach and has been nominated for a variety of awards for her work with parents and children. Paula's passion about ADHD is evident in her talks and portrays and open and honest engagement with her audiences.

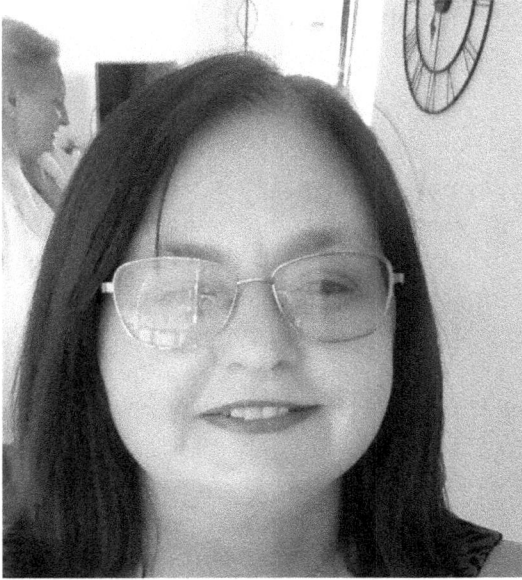

Together We Can Win Any Battle
by Samantha Shepherd

Wow, how life has changed in the last 3.5 years. When I wrote the story for *Parenting A Child on the Spectrum* my life was full of daily dramas, fights, meltdowns and kids that hated their lives. My daughter, then 19, had just been diagnosed with bipolar with schizophrenic tendencies on top of her ASD. She struggled daily with mood swings, anxiety, self-harm thoughts, depression, paranoia and hallucinations. My son, then 16, was diagnosed with Asperger's, experiencing social and separation anxiety, school refusal, depression and recessive language skills. He was determined that he would never be anything, never have any friends, never be able to work, get a girlfriend/wife, have kids or live on his own. He was worried that if he did under some miracle have kids, they would end up like him and go through what he went through, and he never wants anyone to go through what he has been through, not even his worst enemy. He cried regularly and battled depression, anxiety and shutdowns almost daily.

They both often said that they wish they were 'normal' and occasionally wished they weren't here anymore. Getting up and facing the day was hard for them, *and* me. As much as I encouraged, comforted and explained that things would not always be like this and that there was nothing wrong with them and there no such thing as 'normal' as we all are special in our own way, they still struggled. For me, it was a time of heartache, tears, stress, worry and fear. I wondered if I could get both the kids through each day, and at times I struggled to get out of bed in the morning knowing what the day was going to hold. I often worried that one day I would find one of them had taken their own life because they couldn't face another day. I knew I couldn't show my fear, anxieties and tears, as that would just make things worse.

There were many times when I wondered if I was good enough – after all, everyone kept telling me I was doing it all wrong, I needed to be tougher, stricter, use tough love, force them do and face things because if they are not given a choice they would just deal with it. I was told this even by so-called 'professionals', but I stuck to my guns knowing that no-one knows my kids the way I do; they don't live with them, they don't see the daily struggles. I kept parenting with love, understanding, acceptance and patience. Of course, there was discipline, but it was adapted to suit them and never handed out for things that they had little to no control over at the time. I kept appreciating the small things like a smile, a laugh, a hug and the occasional 'I love you, Mum', and that helped on the days that where hard.

Now, 3.5 years later, how things have changed.

Over the years, my daughter, seemed to struggle the most. Well, that is how it would have seemed like to the world; her struggles were more externalised, and she would put herself down and lock herself away into isolation. She used to feel like she was a burden to everyone, and it would be better if she was on her own as she wasn't worth anyone's time or energy. She would lock herself away in her room for days, weeks, even *months* at a time, only coming out of her room for the essentials. No amount of talking or encouragement would change her mind. She thought about suicide, and all different types of self-harm. Things like hand-whaling and stuttering started to become a regular thing when she was at her breaking point. In the previous 19 years she had never stuttered or hand-whaled, so when these signs first appeared they were a big concern, but as time went by we started to consider them a blessing, as then, without her having to say it, I knew when she had had enough. There was no more pushing her beyond her braking point, which meant her thoughts of self-harm went down and we had fewer meltdowns. Don't get me wrong – there was a downside to the stuttering and whaling such as bullies and strangers mocking her, but luckily, 9 times out of 10, she didn't notice, and the other 1 time she learnt to ignore.

My daughter has learnt to make a lot of changes and acceptances over the last 3 years; things we used to dread and avoid she can now attempt or do, and if she can't, she has also learnt to vocalise her inabilities without embarrassment or fear of being ridiculed. Her self-hatred has diminished, and her self-acceptance has grown. We still have bad days, days where she can't get out of bed, days where she cries for no reason, days where she is angry and snappy; but time has taught her to accept these days and, with the help of a loving, patient and tolerant family, she has learnt that she is allowed to have these moods and days, but she isn't allowed to take it out on the rest of us (though this is still a learning process). She is now 22 and has learnt what her own triggers are and the best way to deal with most of them. Yes, she still needs assistance and has a support worker 3 days a week, but she now knows when she is getting close to breaking point to say something, and she always carries with her things that make her feel good and help her stay calm such as squishies, fidgets, music and even one of her teddy bears. She is learning that what makes her different also makes her special, and she is perfect the way she is. She is starting to see what others see in her and rejoice in the likes and her different nature. She is well on her way to learning to love herself and see herself the way others love and see her.

Unlike my daughter, my son's struggles were more internal. I often didn't know when things were wrong or if he was upset as he would keep them to himself so as not to stress or upset me. It is always heartbreaking to know that your child is struggling with everyday things in life such as having friends, wanting a job and, at times, even getting up in the morning, and there was not much you could do about it except encourage, prompt and reassure. But it felt worse knowing he was going through this on his own because he wanted to protect *me*, his Mum. My son has always been a sensitive child that has wanted, and still wants, so many things for himself, and he put so much pressure on himself to be 'normal' – or at least act 'normal' – because he feels that is the only way he will have all the things he wants, i.e. friends to hang out with and to visit or who would visit him, a job, a girlfriend and, in his mind, a future. Many times, I would catch him crying in a corner on his own, the scene was enough to make me want to cry. I would wait until he was calm, and we would talk until he felt a little better, but that didn't stop him for still wanting all those things. No matter how much I reminded him of his achievements and accomplishments he still felt like a failure.

Now, at 19, he has scored himself a job, his dream job, and he loves it. He works 8 hours a week. I know that doesn't sound like much but it's a great start for someone that was unable to leave the house for many years. He loves his job and so looks forward to going in. When I pick him up from work, it's incredible to listen to him ramble on about his day and how proud he is of himself because he did something new, spoke to someone he had never seen before or helped someone find something that they were looking for. The pride on his face is unreal to see. He once said, 'You were right, Mum. You always said I could and would do it, and here I am doing it. It's was a hard road, but so worth it. I'm so proud of myself for not giving up.' It brought tears to my eyes and was probably the one and only time I will *ever* get told I was right about anything! There are still hard times, ups and downs, tears and stress, days where everything gets on top of him, as even doing what he wants – his dream job – is draining and stressful and takes a lot out of him. But he now knows that his daily efforts and internal fights *will* pay off, and he will achieve his dreams if he just keeps moving forward. He now knows that a bad day is just that – one day amongst many – and eventually that bad day will be over, and he can look forward to a new day starting.

I am so proud of my children and all that they have accomplished in the last 3 years. They have pushed themselves (and me, at times) to breaking point, but still managed to achieve great goals. Yes, there always will be struggles, but if you hold on to those achievements it makes those struggles easier to deal with; the light at the end of the tunnel, you could say. I remind them and myself regularly of how things were and how they are now. I tell them every day how proud I am of their achievements. I remind them to be proud of themselves, that they have managed to move forward even in the darkest of times and have brought themselves out of it a stronger person.

I am also proud of myself; I trusted my instincts and thoughts, I ignored the people that said I was doing it wrong and the children wouldn't achieve what they and I wanted if I kept doing the things the way I was, and look at us now!

We are in a town we love (we moved to a small country town, not for everyone but right for us) and the children have achieved great goals and are striving to achieve more. They are very happy and are moving forward at a pace that suits them. They are now making plans for a future that they want, knowing that they can and will achieve them. We have built a fantastically open, honest relationship with each other and they know that they can talk to me about anything. We help support each other through life's ups and downs. It used to only be me, but now we all celebrate the small things in life – a smile, a laugh, a joke, a hug, an 'I love you'. These are things we hold on to, as these things make life worthwhile.

SAMANTHA SHEPHERD *is a mum of 2 young adults, likes to keep busy with work and volunteering at the local historical museum. She loves passing her free time, what little there is, with her friends and family.*

Together We Can Win Any Battle
by Samantha Shepherd

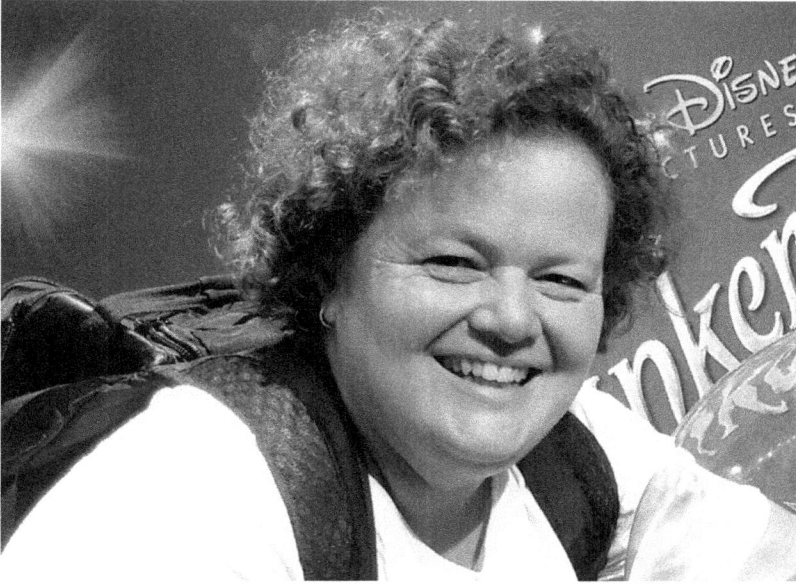

Love, Life, Autism, Tics; Onward We Go!
by Katrina Fowler

Where were we then, in the first instalment, 2015? We were four years into the Autism journey for three out of four of my biological children *and* my ex-husband, the children's father. They had all been diagnosed with Asperger's and Sensory Processing Disorder. Diagnosis for Tim was in 2011, aged 10. Jessica and Michael were diagnosed in 2012, Jessica aged 17.5 and Michael aged 7. It was a whirlwind of chaos and fast learning in how to best manage the boys, who lived with me after I left their dad. Jess and her sisters – Claire, then aged 15, my biological child, and Jess M, also aged 17.5, our long-term foster child, were living with their dad.

At the time of writing the first instalment, Jess was 21, living independently, had attained her Diploma in Children's Services, was working and was engaged.

Claire was boarding with friends and working. Jess M was working, living with Jess and Mike. Tim was thirteen and in high school – mainstream, with support. His transition year had a few hiccups with a few suspensions as he reacted to being bullied and teased. We were actively working in therapy on concepts such as flexible thinking, unexpected events, emotional regulation and getting along with Michael. Michael was ten, in year five at mainstream school with no support but a teacher who understood him. He was my Jekyll and Hyde child, like Jessica, who was great at school and extremely difficult, oppositional and needing to know every detail of every request made of him and every decision made for our family. Therapy for Michael was focused on flexible thinking and getting along with Timothy. Feeling like I was living in a warzone day in and day out was exhausting to say the least.

As I sit to write the second instalment, it is only a few days until 2019 draws to a close. There is the realization that four years have flown by since book one was written. I am writing my chapter for book two, looking back at what has happened in this time, how far my kids have come and of course, wondering what the future will bring in the next four years and beyond.

Let's go back to 2016; Tim was in year 8, Michael in year 6, and both doing well academically. For Tim, high school was still hard as he was the target of bullying, which of course happened out of the sight of teachers. Tim still experienced a couple of suspensions as he reacted to the bullying. He was never an instigator, but violence in public schools results in suspension. He has less suspensions than year seven, so he was learning to self-regulate and trying so hard to ignore the bullies. He was able to attend the safe space of learning support when he needed and often went there at break time as it was quiet and monitored. Tim had built a fantastic relationship with learning support. Learning support really understood how Tim 'worked', as did many of his teachers. The decision to move to be able to attend this school was really paying off. I felt that I too had a good working relationship with the Learning Support Team, and we worked together for Tim. The biggest challenge for Tim was assessments, where every time he received one, he would not be able to function and think through what had to be done. His brain froze and he said he did not know what to do and did not know any answers. This happened without fail for every assessment he received, resulting in grumbling, opposition, avoidance and hating school. Every assessment required me to read the assessment task, reword and ask him the questions that the task was asking and then being able to say, 'See? You *do* know it, Tim.' Every assessment, after this beginning process, required me to sit and work with him to help him structure and write the assessment. I tried to use each assessment to encourage him in planning and preparation, breaking it down into smaller steps and finding relevant information for him to read and ask him about what he read. Had this worked now that we are in 2019 and year 11? Yes, there is an increase in his ability to do assessments without me sitting with him for every question.

Michael continued to be a chatterbox at school but had a teacher who also 'got' him and quickly learnt that it didn't matter where he sat Michael, he would chat! He kept Michael seated where he would be the least distracted and with whom he worked well with. Michael was very social at school and played soccer and handball. He, too, had to have the rules followed by everyone and would be vocal if someone did not. This did not seem to cause issues. 2016 also saw Michael return to soccer for the first time since our move in 2014. I signed him up to a local team to where we lived, and not to a team where the primary school was zoned. Soccer provided him with the opportunity to learn to play in a team and learn about how to be a good teammate and demonstrate good sportsmanship. It also introduced him to boys who would be entering high school with him in 2017. The end of primary school was largely uneventful for Michael and he loved his end of year formal. He meandered through school on his own terms and life at home continued to be full of opposition, negotiating, asking a hundred and one questions as he needed to know every detail about anything and everything. He was very demand avoidant and trying to work to a schedule was a continual battle.

2017 was the year that I felt like the worst parent on earth. I felt gutted, useless and like a hopeless parent. I felt like I had failed my son and had not given him enough time in teaching him about Autism, emotions, attending therapy and failed at recognizing his needs as I had been so caught up in managing his brother.

2017 was high school for Michael. He had a few familiar faces due to soccer and some familiarity of the place due to transition days. Michael was known to Learning Support, but he did not have funding from the Department of Education as did Tim. Although both boys have the same diagnosis of Asperger's and Sensory Processing Disorder, they are so very different as evidenced by their reassessment diagnosis under the DSM-V, where Michael had been diagnosed Autism Spectrum Disorder Level 1 and Tim Level 2. Under DSM-V Asperger's no longer exists, but they will always be my Aspie-boys, and Jess my Aspergirl. Although Michael had no funding, I knew that Learning Support would be there if needed.

So, back to year 7 for Michael. Term one went so smoothly, and I was so surprised at how well he adapted to high school. He would even ask Tim any questions that were school related as Tim was now in his third year at high school. The boys communicated and worked together! For Tim, year 9 was where the classes were graded, and he left behind the bullies as he was put in the top classes for Math and Science. Life at school was still a challenge but he was doing well socially and academically. In regard to his behaviour, he had only one warning all year! Again, this was in reaction to being bullied. Socially, he had made friends who played the same card games as he did. Many afternoons after school saw our dining table filled with teen boys and their cards and snacks of course. At the end of the year, I had planned a surprise birthday party for Tim and his friends at an escape room. They had a great time.

Term two for Michael saw the unravelling of a smooth transition into high school and the rise of tics, rages and sensory overload. Michael was still playing soccer and the time to get ready for soccer was much more than expected for any regular teen due to how his socks and shin pads had to go on and feel *just right* before his boots could go on, and be just the right tension when done up.

This was not a new happening, but it was beginning to take longer and longer, and my frustration levels rose each training night and game day. Little did I know what was to come!

School was beginning to be impacted by the sensory issues and it was taking longer and longer for Michael to get socks and shoes on his feet. My confident, happy young man was changing, and both his motor and vocal tics were evident and impacting his ability to get ready for school in addition to the sensory issues he was experiencing. The challenge was that I did not know as this was happening that it was likely a hormonal flood giving rise to the behaviours I was seeing. Anytime in the past that I had raised the issues of tics and obsessive behaviours, I was told it was just part of Autism. Michael arrived later and later to school as mornings saw him raging and punching his feet, yelling how stupid his feet were, saying they needed to be cut off and how he wished he did not have feet. He would throw his shoes and socks, cry and scream and go to his room. His days at school got shorter and his attendance dropped. We had negotiated wearing slippers to school and only having his joggers on to attend classes such as cooking and woodwork. If he couldn't attend class, he could go to Learning Support. This lasted a few weeks until he was no longer at school as I had decided that school was not worth what it was doing to my boy. School was not worth him being miserable and hating himself, his body and wanting to harm himself. Michael could no longer get socks and shoes on his feet and I was not going to push him to achieve this. I hated every day that I witnessed him yelling, screaming, punching and hating himself. What had happened and what had I missed for us to get to this? I had meeting with Learning support and the deputy principal and was able to negotiate that work was sent home and we schooled at home, when we could, so that he did not lag behind academically.

By term three, Michael was at home full time, schooling at home and the next meeting at school was to discuss transitioning him to Distance Education. Soccer, like school, was now a non-event. During the time of decreasing attendance to soccer, the coach was so encouraging and inclusive of Michael. He ensured Michael did have game time when he was able to play, and he ensured he provided Michael with praise and encouragement. Sadly, Michael could not play out the season due to not being able to get shin pads, socks and boots on his feet. He was even convinced he was a bad player, which he was not. Term three also saw us attending two Occupational Therapists, a Music Therapist and a Psychologist weekly as well as consulting a Behaviour Therapist, Podiatrist and Chiropractor. At home it was a challenge to get Michael to do schoolwork and he spent many hours in his room, under his covers. He did not engage much with the therapists and did not want to be at any of the sessions. I was defeated and felt scared for his future, for *our* future, and thought that I had lost my boy to whatever was going on, as no one had an answer for us! It was a year later, when talking to a friend about what had happened, that I sent her videos of the events, that she suggested that it may indeed be Tourette Rages, known for sudden onset in puberty. Whilst we have sought a paediatrician, the diagnosis has returned as Childhood Tic Disorder, although he does fall under the criteria for Tourette's. We have also since seen a psychologist as per requirements for insurance funding and she totally dismissed the Tic Disorder diagnosis, blaming the Autism diagnosis. We have so far been refused requests for a referral to a Paediatric Neurologist.

Term four of 2017 saw Michael return to school four days a week. He got to choose what days he would go, according to his timetable. Therapy took a back seat to school as per Michael's request and we fitted in what we could after school. 2018 saw Michael return to school full time, of his own accord, and we haven't looked back! He continues to do very well academically and found his place amongst his peers. This year, 2019, he has chosen music production and cross-fit for electives. He is attending supported music lessons for the guitar weekly as his only therapy input and has started dating a lovely young lady in term four. At school, he is part of a year 9 rock band and they have performed on numerous occasions. He has also had a few vocal lessons to be able to sing in the band, and hopefully will continue to explore this avenue.

2018 was year 10 for Tim, and he continued to do well academically and had no incidents regarding behaviour. He had learnt to self-regulate; he could now understand sarcasm and that in his world of black and white there is a lot of grey, which is where most people operate. His gaming friends had gone to senior school and he was establishing new friendships both in and out of gaming. For his year 10 formal, I had made his tie from fabric of the Periodic Table, and his science teachers loved it and wanted one, too! A few days before formal, he was invited by a lovely young lady to go with her in her uncle's vintage car. I was more excited by the car than Tim! He decided to go, and they recently celebrated one year of dating! The highlight of Tim's Year 10 year was the award assembly at the end of the year. Tim was awarded The Phoenix Award. 'For your perseverance, hard work and efforts to overcome. May you rise from the ashes and above the challenges that life throws your way.' I remember running up to the Learning Support teacher after the assemble and crying, 'We did it, he did it, he made it!'

This year, 2019, saw Tim move over to senior school and to a whole set of new challenges and changes. The support from Learning Support is less than ideal and does nothing but frustrate him, despite what seemed to be promised as he came to senior school with funding for support. My frustration at senior school has had me considering removing him from school because he was 17 at the beginning of year 11. A few, lovely, understanding teachers have reminded me that school is worth it for Tim, at this point in time. At the end of 2019, he has achieved a Certificate 3 in Aviation: Line of Sight Drone Pilot Licence, and also finished his Certificate 2 in Metals and Engineering, a VET course, including sitting the HSC exam for this subject. He does not want to be at school anymore and we have had discussions with the Careers teacher about ongoing work experience or work placement for his year 12 year, to also allow him to finish Engineering Studies as he does not yet have any employment. I do not want him at home doing nothing as I hope the Engineering Studies provides him with more areas of interest that he can consider for his future pathways.

Last, but definitely not least, my girls – where are they now?

Jessica, my Aspergirl, eloped with her fiancé in Las Vegas, dressed as Wonder Woman and Superman, in February 2017. They announced their marriage with a photo on Facebook. While I wasn't totally surprised, I was sad that I did not get to be at my daughter's wedding. I was super excited when I realized the Superman cape that Mike wore was the one that I had made for him, at their request for a party, so they told me. We celebrated with a small wedding photo shoot so they could wear the wedding dress and suit they already had, and a reception when they got home where Jessica had to help me with making and decorating their cake as I had broken my wrist. In 2018, Jess and Mike packed their bags and left for the United Kingdom on an Ancestry visa to work and travel. As the end of 2019 draws near, they have made their way in the world, Mike working on the rails as was always his dream and Jessica having left childcare to work on the rails too. We talk most days and do lots of video calls as well. They have also purchased their own two-bedroom unit. They are taking every opportunity to travel and see more of the world, too.

Claire, my only neurotypical biological daughter, has found her place in the world too. This year she gained an electrical apprenticeship and is enjoying her new life choice away from home, aged and disability care, where she had been since the first instalment. She has become a strong and independent young lady in her own right. She visits regularly and has a great relationship with her brothers and me. I think we have done a lot of healing and gained a better understanding of each other.

Jess M, my long-term foster daughter, moved to be closer to me in 2018. It has been wonderful seeing her grow into a capable young lady. We were blessed this year with a beautiful surprise package of a granddaughter. Miss Ruby is our first grandchild, and she is adored by all and doted on by her uncles and aunts who are all very capable of looking after her and attending her needs. As I had said in the first book – if Autism was to be in our future, then I feel prepared to be able to be pro-active in support and education where it is needed. And it may be needed, as Ruby's dad has Asperger's and learning difficulties, as does Jess M. Ruby already has her first weighted blanket and has grown so much that she probably needs an upgrade now! She responds well to lavender oil (diluted of course) to help her little body relax, and she loves lavender soap in her bath. At eleven weeks old, she is regularly sleeping six to seven hours at night, which has helped her dad manage better and of course helped Jess feel better, too.

We have had an eventful few years. As for myself, in 2017 I broke my wrist, so the boys had to step up and be more self-sufficient and independent. In 2018, my partner and I went on the European River Cruise while the boys stayed at their dad's. It was the trip of a lifetime, and so relaxing yet busy. I was blessed that Jessica and Mike could take the time to come and meet us in Amsterdam at the end of our cruise. We had a lovely three days together. In 2019, I was able to fulfill my lifelong wish and hope and have a breast reduction. At 51 years of age I thought maybe it was too late, and never knew until twelve months prior, due to waiting time for accessibility for private health insurance, that the journey could be an actual reality. The post-surgery restrictions again meant that they boys had to step up and be more responsible for the day to day events of living: cooking, cleaning, dishes and laundry. Important life skills, I reminded them when they would complain. Having the surgery was the best decision I have ever made regarding my own self-care. I urge you to not always put yourself last!

And what for our future? We have a trip planned to the UK for February 2020. The boys have never been on an international flight before and neither has Jess M. There are six of us going, with baby Ruby, of course. We have a little over two weeks to spend with Jessica and Mike and I am counting down the days now!

What message would I leave you with? Hope, Faith and Love. Believe in yourself, trust yourself and care for yourself. You never know what might cross your path and bring light to your darkness. It is not always an easy ride and different ages have their own challenges. Aim high and accept where you are for now. Tomorrow is a new day. Sending love, light and blessings to you!

KATRINA FOWLER *is a mum of five, with three diagnosed on the Autism Spectrum (Asperger's, one being my Aspergirl). Grandma to one. Two teen boys at home now, the girls have flown the coop. She is studying to re-enter the workforce and volunteer her time with mentoring, teaching sewing or sewing for herself and charity.*

Love, Life, Autism, Tics; Onward We Go!
by Katrina Fowler

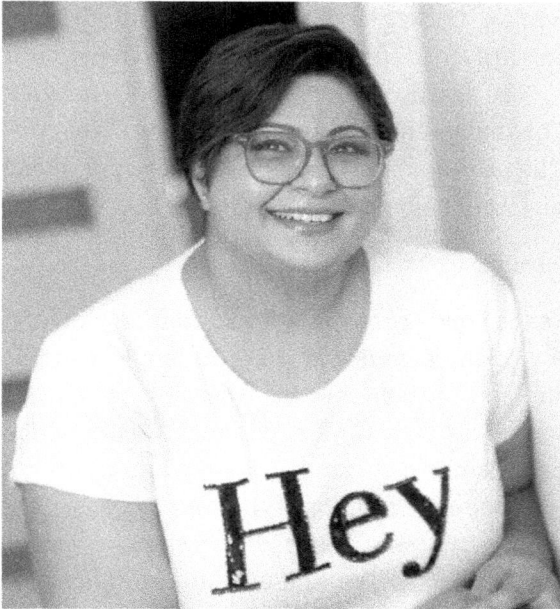

Be Brave
by Cindy Corrie

Well, the last three years have been the biggest in my life. Like many families of children on the Autism spectrum, we found that there wasn't an educational option that embraced their unique perspectives and strengths and supported them to work towards developmental goals. I started to hear about the very scary statistics around independence and employment for people on the Autism spectrum, and frankly, I thought that those outcomes were not acceptable.

I was a corporate insurance broker at the time, and I was filling in for a colleague who looked after independent schools. I took the opportunity to put myself out there and meet with the executive director at the peak association for independent schools in Queensland. I walked into his office and told him about our predicament with schooling options. Unfortunately, he didn't reveal any hidden treasure. 'You could open your own school,' he said with a chuckle. Open a school? The thought hadn't crossed my mind at that point. I asked about the process and he gave me a huge wad of paperwork. 'Read that, and if we ever see you again, we'll help you open a school.'

We opened the school.

We spent weekends holding community forums in public libraries all over Brisbane, listening to the experiences of local families and hearing what was important to them and to their children when it came to school experiences. What I learned the most from that experience was how diverse our Autism community is. Each family came from varying backgrounds and had varying experiences, which made the process of community consultation so important. We started to understand more about what Sycamore was going to look like, what the culture needed to be like, and what the staff needed to embody.

By this time, the community demand was growing, and we had nearly 500 expressions of interest in enrolment for the school. Using the data we collected, we discovered that the Redlands area of Brisbane not only had a number of families looking for support, but also lacked many of the wrap-around services the Autism community needed to provide holistic support to their children. And then a most serendipitous journey ensued...

At a business forum breakfast, I met a lady from a government department that managed state owned assets. She introduced herself and asked me who I was. I said, 'I'm Cindy Corrie, and I'm working to open a school for children with Autism.' Usually when I tell people this, I get the 'she's dreaming' look, but this woman was actually intrigued. She asked me where the school was going to be and I said that so far, we're looking at the Redlands area as a possible site for the first catchment. 'There are so many unused government assets out here. I'm going to put you in touch with someone at the local council who might be able to help you out.' I was grateful, but not hopeful that anything would come from the conversation. Then, a couple of weeks later, I received a call from a man named Doug Hunt at Redland City Council. I started my usual spiel: 'I'm working to open a school for kids on the Autism spectrum because there's a huge community in need for educational parity and tailored learning environments…' I was interrupted with, 'Oh, I've got four kids, two of which are on the spectrum, so I know exactly where you're coming from.' My shoulders just dropped, and I took a huge breath and thought, 'Thank God, someone I actually need support from understands personally why I'm doing this!'

Within a week Doug and I met, and a few days later I was walking around what would be the home of The Sycamore School. It was a run-down building at the back of the local vocational education campus, and within a few months, we got the final tick from the state government to open our school.

Once we were granted accreditation to open The Sycamore School, I dropped *everything* to get that school open. I had a very short six months before the new school year. I quit my job and went full speed ahead, pouring everything I had into ensuring we could support as many kids as possible by the beginning of the school year. By this time, we'd had a clearer vision about what the school would provide and considered the many stories we'd learned in speaking with the wider community in our community forums, which we held on weekends when we weren't holding fundraising events. But I needed more than sausage sizzles to get the funds I needed not only to open the school, but to pay for the operating costs for the first six months until government funding started to trickle in. I needed a rich person to give me money… and FAST!

I started attending events for start-ups. Most of them were tech companies, but what astounded me was the number of people who were committed to see social benefits of their investments. Philanthropists and investors alike were driven by positive outcomes, and I knew, this was my key to funding our school. I started approaching social impact intermediaries and found one that really believed in the changes we could make if Sycamore existed. They supported us to build our financial model and held an event for investors to attend and hear our story. Our intermediary was based in Sydney, and I waited with bated breath for a phone call from the intermediary to hear about the outcome of their event, and I was overwhelmed with excitement and relief that a syndicate of investors had pitched in to fund our start-up. It was an incredibly exciting time. And a very stressful time...

The weight of the work ahead started to bear down, and I questioned my ability to get this over the finish line. In the meantime, we'd appointed a Principal, and began working through enrolments, staff recruitment, financial processes, compliance processes... you name it! We worked 24/7 for months.

Meeting our students and starting to understand the impact of the mere existence of our school was the biggest motivation for me to keep going. I met families and children who had been completely disengaged from education for years, students who had been severely bullied, parents who had given up their careers because their children were excluded from school so frequently. But their hope kept me going. Their belief in me and what this school could provide made me more tenacious each day. We started to hear from the children how much they looked forward to going to a school where all their friends were 'just like me', 'liked the same things', and relief they had about not being 'the different one'. For me, there was one word that summed up what they were looking for... **INCLUSION**!

INCLUSION – probably the most controversial word in the Autism community. Typically, inclusion means all children of all abilities and disabilities learning in the same classroom with age-appropriate typically developing peers. And while the value of this is undoubtedly beneficial, it only accounts for equality – not equity. Equality is limited – it provides the SAME access, levels of support, learning environments and methods of delivery as every other student. Equity is what we're really striving for – where each student is provided with the level of support that is required to meet their needs, regardless of whether they are developmental or academic. And this is EXACTLY what we wanted to ensure at

Be Brave
by Cindy Corrie

The Sycamore School – that EVERY STUDENT is provided with the necessary supports to help them achieve their personal goals.

Finally, our school opened on the 23rd January 2017 to 44 students. We've now grown to 92 students from prep to Year 9, most of whom live locally. We have made an incredible impact on their academic progress and their developmental progress with a focus on positive emotional intelligence building, reflective practice and developing skills in self-advocacy and self-determination – to support independence in decision making later in life. We NEVER suspend or expel – we take ownership of our behaviour and accept that learning to use our strategies supports everyone. Our school community is now supported, with access to a multi-disciplinary team who support students at school, and support families equally. The ripple effects this educational option has had on the family life of our students is immeasurable. Their relationships with their parents and siblings have flourished, their home lives are more functional and independent, and their parents are re-engaged in employment. Families have moved from interstate and overseas to attend The Sycamore School, and we continue to work towards supporting more students in the future.

Sycamore is doing something about the educational disparity students with Autism experience. It provides an opportunity to learn the things about our world that typically developing kids learn through osmosis, but that we need to explicitly teach – emotional intelligence, communication, sensory regulation, social communication and behavioural support. Alongside all these things, our students learn the national curriculum like every other student in the country.

We've now got an educational setting that not only teaches our kids the things they can't learn through osmosis like other kids, but a school that gives them an opportunity to have educational parity, to have positive schooling experiences, to have meaningful friendships, to be confident self-advocates, to have opportunities to change their predicted futures, to mend broken families, and most of all, to have a sense of belonging and feel included. The things that all children have a right to experience.

We teach our kids at Sycamore that Autism is their superpower – that they embody unique perspectives that others don't. And that they should be proud of the incredible things they do, regardless of how brave they had to be to get there.

2018 saw further development and a bedding-down of our model at The Sycamore School, and my role became more strategic, working to support our Autism community more broadly. I enjoyed still being able to contribute to the Autism community this way and had a very supportive Board and Principal. But during 2018, I faced my biggest challenge yet...

We'd decided in the July school holidays of that year to make our annual family pilgrimage to the Sunshine Coast to take Joseph to the Zoo and Aquarium. Busily packing for our trip, I accidently tripped and caught myself from falling on the bathroom door frame. I had bumped my chest in the breast area, and it didn't feel like the soft landing I expected. I felt this hardened area on my breast, and I thought that maybe I had been left with a bruise or bump from the fall. Thinking nothing of it, we continued to pack and made our way to the Sunshine Coast. While we were away, I couldn't help but keep feeling the bump from the fall and in the back of my mind, I thought, 'this isn't normal.' I went to see my husband in the bedroom... 'I think I've done something to my breast when I fell the other day... unless this lump was already there?' It actually hadn't crossed my mind that the lump may have been there before the fall. I panicked. My husband, being the less neurotic person in the relationship, said 'Don't jump to conclusions. Go and see the GP when we get home... and stop thinking about it.'

We arrived back home a couple of days later, and I made an appointment to see the GP. I waited in the waiting room, until she called me in. We entered the examination room, and I sat down on the chair next to her desk. 'What's going on?' she asked. I said, 'I think I've found a lump on my right breast. It could be from a fall but, I'm not sure.' She asked me to lay down on the examination bed in the room and examined my breasts. Nothing went through my mind, I just laid there waiting for her to tell me what was going on. 'Sit up for me,' she eventually said. 'There's definitely a large lump in your right breast, and I think you need to get to a diagnostic clinic urgently. I'm gonna call them now and get you an appointment tomorrow.' I said, 'I can't go tomorrow, I have a fundraiser at the school tomorrow, and I need to be there.' She made me an appointment for a couple of days' time… Friday.

I left the doctor's office and called my husband straight away. He reassured me there's nothing to worry about… until there's something to worry about. It annoyed me how calm he was, but I knew he was right. I said, 'It's going to take most of the day – what about Joseph? We need to pick him up from school, and I need you with me at the clinic.'

We agreed I would call my mother to see if she could help. My mother works with my father in their mortgage broking business. I called her. 'Are you in your office? Can you close the door?' There was a pause. 'What's going on?' she asked. I replied, 'So I've just been to the GP, and they've found a lump in my right breast, and I need to go to the diagnostic clinic on Friday so could you please pick Joseph up from school?'

There was this deafening silence.

'Shit Cindy! Shit!' she said softly.

I could tell she was crying. I said that we didn't know what it is yet and we shouldn't jump to conclusions. I asked her to tell my father when she thought it was an appropriate time, since they were at work. I asked her to tell my sister and brother also – I didn't have it in me to repeat what I had just said. She agreed and said that she would pick Joseph up for me on Friday afternoon.

Friday came. We took Joseph to before-school care and made our way to the clinic. The great thing about this clinic is that they can provide you with a diagnosis in 24 hours, and while it was an expensive option, I couldn't imagine having to wait days for what could be life-changing news. They dressed me in a gown, gave me a cup of tea, and part of me felt this was their way of softening some kind of blow! My head was empty. Not a thought went through my mind, I was just totally present – it was a surreal experience. I had a mammogram and an ultrasound on my breasts, and then I waited with my husband to be seen by a diagnostics doctor. Finally, the doctor called both my husband and me into her office.

'So, there's a four-centimetre tumour (about the size of a golf-ball) and a two-and-a-half-centimetre tumour (about the size of a marble) in your right breast. Unfortunately, they look suspicious and I'd like to take a biopsy of both tumours and a lymph node so we can get some more information about them.'

We went through the motions – I had biopsies of the tumours and lymph node done right there and then in the clinic, using big needles that they placed in my breast to extract samples for testing. Once it was over, the doctor told me she would send these for urgent testing and give me a call on Monday and let me know the outcome. We left the clinic and made our way to mum and dad's place where they had picked up Joseph. We told them everything that happened in the clinic. My sister and brother joined us when they finished work. We have a family tradition – when the going gets tough for someone in our family, we all congregate at mum and dad's, and dad makes cocktails for everyone. We spend out toughest times together drinking cocktails, and this night was possibly the hardest we all had ever faced. Everyone was trying to be optimistic and positive. They kept telling me there was nothing to worry about, I didn't have any of the risk factors, I was too young, and that everything would be fine. I went along with it to ease their anxieties... but deep down I was preparing for the worst.

Over the weekend, I tried to keep life as normal as possible. In my mind, I was fighting off the 'dark place' we all go to when we're faced with impossible challenges. I just waited for Monday – and it couldn't come soon enough.

I remember I was walking around in the local chemist to buy more dressings for my biopsy wounds when my phone rang. I'd been expecting a call from the doctor with the results of the biopsies. I answered the phone...

'Cindy speaking.'

'Hi, Cindy. It's Doctor Belinda Stevens from the clinic, how are you?'

'Ok, thanks.'

'I wanted to let you know the results of the biopsies we took on Friday are back.'

It felt like the whole world stopped turning at this moment. Her pause felt like hours...

'... Unfortunately, both of those tumours are malignant. I'm sorry. I'm referring you to a breast surgeon who may want to run some further tests, but it's important that you make an appointment to see the surgeon as soon as possible. They will discuss treatment options with you. I'm sorry for the bad news.'

I knew it. I just *knew* it. Something in me knew all along this was going to be where it landed. I left the chemist and went back to my office at the school. I closed the door, called my husband and told him the news.

This wasn't our first rodeo. In 2012, about a month before Joseph was diagnosed with Autism, I was diagnosed with Multiple Sclerosis. Luckily, since then my MS has been pretty dormant, and I'd been off treatment for a couple of years. So, we'd been through what we thought was our share of dealing with bad news and facing difficult challenges – but it seemed that wasn't the case. When I told my husband that the tumours were malignant, his response was, 'Why not?' It had almost become like we should just accept that these things will happen to us. My parents and siblings through the weekend had been researching on Google and had convinced themselves that I was going to be fine. When I told them the tumours were malignant, they were devastated. And while I knew deep down this was going to be the result, I couldn't believe that I had cancer.

There, I said it... the C-word. I had Cancer. I was 36 years old and I had *Cancer*.

Immediately, my concern was Joseph and how I was going to support him through this journey, though I didn't know what the journey would entail. In that time, we told our school community, which was a very difficult thing to do, but we did it because we needed their support in helping Joseph through this process. We had a meeting with his education team and therapists, and they worked together to write Joseph a book about cancer. We called it The Evil Germ. Chemotherapy was called Superjuice, and the story line was that mummy would take Superjuice at the hospital to help her fight the evil germ. And the harder she fought, the more she would change. She would become more tired, she would lose her hair, she wouldn't be able to do all the things she would normally do, but she would keep everything the same for Joseph. We worked very hard to keep routines as normal as possible. My sister moved in part-time and cooked healthy meals for me (if I could stomach them), and the whole family banded together and helped with school pick-ups. We had a plan in place!

I saw the surgeon a couple of days later, and he confirmed worse news. I had Triple Negative Breast Cancer (TNBC) – a rare breast cancer that was difficult to treat and had a high chance of recurrence.

GREAT! I HAD TO GET THE RARE ONE! The surgeon told us that TNBC is best treated with chemotherapy first to shrink the tumours, then surgery following that. He referred me to an oncologist, and the oncologist saw me within the week.

From the day I received the dreaded phone call from the diagnostic doctor, it was what seemed like a very quick two weeks, and I was due to start chemotherapy.

Part of having intravenous chemo is a risk to the health of your veins, and veins are important if you're having chemo intravenously! So, they put a port-a-cath in your chest to administer the chemo with – it's a plastic device about the size of a soft-drink bottle lid that is inserted in your chest. Attached to the port is a catheter that is fed through a vein near your collarbone and down into a main vein near the heart. On my first day of chemo, I had surgery to have the port inserted in the morning, and in the afternoon, I had my first dose of chemo... that was a hard, hard day! The anxiety around having surgery is one thing, but knowing I was going to have chemo later that day was another. I came through relatively unscathed and didn't feel the effects of chemo so much that day.

Cancer treatment was a long, *long* journey, and it took everything in me to commit myself to it. I (unlike people with a hint of sanity) continued to work part-time during all of my treatment. I endured one of the worst kinds of chemotherapy – eight weeks (four fortnightly doses) of a chemo so bad they call it The Red Devil. I lost my hair, eyebrows and eyelashes, I suffered from severe anaemia, I had to have blood transfusions... it was a tough ride. Following that course of chemotherapy, I had to get through a 12-week course (a dose each week) of another chemotherapy called Taxol. It was also intravenous. I'd come to terms with being on chemo and the energy it takes from you, but I was so nervous about how I was going to cope doing a dose every week. A week is so short, and it felt like all the weeks just rolled together. But it was about to become even more eventful... we learned I was a *one percent-er*...

Every Tuesday was chemo day, and each Tuesday my family would spend it with me at the hospital while I had chemo (which would take all day), and then we would all meet at mum and dads for dinner afterwards. One Tuesday, it was time for the fifth dose of Taxol. I was all hooked up and ready to go, the nurse hit the button to start the treatment, and all of a sudden, I started to feel different. My body felt like it was on fire, my heart was beating very fast, my skin was burning, my breathing was short and fast... I hit the nurse call button. They came running in and immediately stopped the treatment. As soon as the treatment stopped, my symptoms started to subside – I'd had an allergic reaction to Taxol. I WAS ALLERGIC TO CHEMO!! The nurse called my oncologist...

'So, Cindy has had a reaction to Taxol on her fifth dose...'

'Of course, she has! She's my one percent-er! She gets the rare cancer and the rare treatment side effects!'

Don't get me wrong I love feeling special, but this was just going too far. It meant that to get through the next eight doses, I would have to have high doses of steroids and antihistamines, as well as a slower administration of the drug. Great – chemo was going to take longer, and I was going to have to take more drugs to get through it!

It worked, and I continued treatment, but the steroids would keep me up for *days* after chemo. I had so much energy and stayed up all night watching movies *and* working! Eventually, my MS caught up with me and interfered with my chemo treatment, and I managed to get through 10 out of the 12 doses of Taxol. Following Taxol, I endured three surgeries to remove the residual cancer that chemo didn't kill (it took the surgeon three attempts before he could get it all out! – just me being special again) and six weeks of daily radiation. Following that, I did another six months of oral chemotherapy, and finally finished treatment in November 2019. It took 486 days – I was counting!

What got me through all this was the great examples Joseph and all our Sycamore students set for me. There were days when I refused to go to hospital for treatment, I cried every night in the shower, I hated myself for getting sick, I hated the way I looked. I was bald and I hated being bald… and if one more person told me 'it's just hair' I was going to chase them with a pair of clippers and shave *their* head! I didn't know the person who was staring at me in the mirror. I was very, *very* worried about the future. But Joseph has shown me for years how to be brave. For Joseph to live in a world that was so challenging and almost foreign to him and to try and overcome those challenges took so much courage. And if he's going to put in the effort, then so was I. This kept my perspective in check. I continued to measure all things on the effort our children on the Autism spectrum put into achieving things that are innately so difficult for them.

Be Brave

by Cindy Corrie

So, my tip is to be BRAVE. Be brave like you have to speak when you can't. Be brave like you have to look at someone's face even though their expressions seem so puzzling. Have the courage to be around so much busyness and noise, even if it makes you want to flee. Be strong enough to ask for help when the world overwhelms you.

Be PROUD to share what makes you unique. Great minds DON'T think alike... and thank goodness for that!

CINDY CORRIE: *Parent to a child on the Autism Spectrum, advocate, speaker, and founder of The Sycamore School for children with Autism. Cindy has dedicated her time to improving diversity and inclusion in our communities and was awarded an Australia Day Local Hero Award for her work in 2018. Cindy's mission now is to support organisations on their journeys toward true inclusion.*

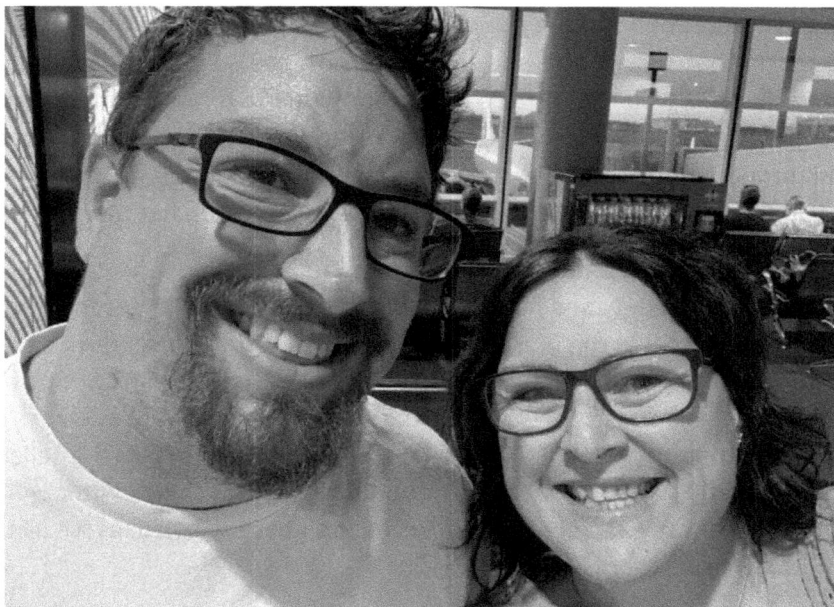

The Journey Continues
by Paul & Rachael Rendle

A quick recap on our story:

We are Paul and Rachael Rendle, and we have three children; Thea, now aged eleven, Oisin, now aged eight, and Oscar, now aged six. Thea and Oisin are both Autistic, and Thea also has Cerebral Palsy Right Hemiplegia.

In *Our Journey So Far*, our chapter in the first *Parenting A Child on the Spectrum*, we detailed Oisin's anxiety and managing him attending an ECDP, and Thea attending a mainstream school and struggling with her anxiety.

Firstly, let's start with Oisin. He went through two Early Childhood Development Programs and had a delayed entry for his prep year at school. Fortunately, we managed to enrol him into a mainstream school that had a MAC unit (Multi Aged Class) that was specialised in children on the spectrum. We had also decided that this would be Thea's new school. Due to a lack of understanding on her previous school principal's & HOSE (Head of Special Education)'s part on how to properly support a child with a complex duel diagnosis, Thea did not get the support that she needed. This had an adverse effect on her mental health.

Unfortunately, Oisin did not adapt well to the full days in the MAC units entry class. Due to his anxiety and not being able to engage with his teacher, he was put on half days within the first couple of weeks of term one. By term 2 he was reviewed by the Guidance Officer for the school as he was constantly bolting and destroying his classrooms. We got the report back a couple of weeks prior to the end of term two that Oisin had been verified with an intellectual impairment and would qualify to attend a special school. Although the verification did come as a shock to us, we needn't have worried, as we all fell in love with his new school on the first visit.

So, with a lot of going back and forth, Oisin was finally able to start at the local special school at the beginning of term 3 for his prep year. Almost immediately we saw a change in him. He was actually having fun and would tell us how great his school was. By the third day at the school he was on the school transport bus, and off he went. There was no looking back, and now he's at a point we thought would never come – he's learning and enjoying himself. Of course, there have been a few bumps in the road, mostly to do with his climbing antics that have led to a few rather amusing tales coming from the school, including tree climbing and egging the principal on to get him, or the time he climbed a fence in to a neighbour's back garden and was promptly returned back with a 'Does this belong to you?' Saying that though, he does love the school and the teachers. Even now, his reward for a good week is to see his first teacher there (which she has no complaints about).

Thea started her year 3 at the MAC unit in her new school, and we started seeing a change in her. She was no longer fighting to use her iPad for writing;

she was enjoying herself and making friends. Her teacher was phenomenal, she had done what no one else could – she had gotten Thea to *want* to be at school, and she was enjoying herself.

Thea breezed through years 3 and 4. Unfortunately, it wasn't to last. Coming towards the end of last year, the school announced that there would be changes. Our HoSE was transferred, and we were given a replacement. We also got a new principal, who was rapidly followed by the department's new inclusion policy. This is when everything went downhill incredibly quickly. Our introduction to the new leadership team at the school was a quick 'Hello', which was then followed by a bombshell; the MAC unit will be closed down from next year as the department will no longer allow it to be in operation. There were lots of meetings with the parents, information sharing and one-on-one discussions with the Head of Inclusion (the new name for the HoSE). To say we were devastated for Thea and panicking is putting it mildly. Thea had tried mainstream and it didn't work. At the end of her year 2 she was physically and mentally drained. We were determined that that wouldn't happen to her again.

The information provided to us from the school was outdated. The inclusion officer gave us handouts with data sourced from a Harvard professor from the '90s. He stated how great inclusive education was for all children on the spectrum (this same professor went on to become an advisor to President Bush). It took us 30 minutes of Google research to find information from *Australia* in *this* decade about the pros and cons for inclusive education for children on the spectrum.

To be clear, we do not think that all children on the spectrum should be excluded from mainstream. We know that there are Autistic children in mainstream classes and that they're thriving. However, there are also those that cannot manage a mainstream setup but don't qualify for a Special School – this is where Thea falls. Not all neurotypical children are the same; equally, not all neurodiverse/Autistic children are the same.

Unfortunately, we don't think the Department of Education sees it the same way. We believe they see it as ASD or non-ASD. Also, the school did not see a problem in putting the responsibility onto the mainstream children to support the MAC children. We were told that the mainstream children would give our children 'wings to fly' and would be encouraging them every step of the way. This was in spite of the fact that there had been no proper introductions or transitions between the different classes.

Before Thea even started her year 5, we went through everything we could with the school. Specific arrangements and support plans for Thea were promised for day one. The new school year started; Oisin was off on the bus from day one to his school, Oscar (our baby from the previous book) was starting his prep year, and Thea was off to her new year and new setup. Unfortunately for her, it was a disaster. By the end of the first week, nothing that we had agreed on had been done. The Head of Inclusion was not doing her job, and within a couple of weeks she had left to go on maternity leave. A replacement was brought in who had no idea about Thea and her complex needs as there had been *zero* handover. What the school forgot – or just didn't care about – was that when Thea started at this school she was traumatised and had severe trust issues after her year 2 in her previous school. Her teacher in the MAC unit worked incredibly hard with her. She gained Thea's trust and rebuilt her confidence. Thea was missing her and her classmates desperately. She felt safe in her MAC classroom and couldn't understand why it had been closed and why she couldn't have her adored teacher anymore.

The school was in a mess. There was no communication between the principal and her staff, and there had been no proper transition for the children to come out of the MAC unit into mainstream. Our suspicions were confirmed – this was the hardest year of Thea's schooling to date.

By the end of term 1, we were struggling daily to get her in to school. Constant phone calls were made to the school trying to get them to listen to what was happening. We emailed them letters from Thea's psychiatrist warning them of the damage to her mental health if they didn't get it right. Unfortunately, it all fell on deaf ears; as far as they were concerned, they knew what was best, and they started making decisions without telling us. For example, Thea handled staying in a mainstream class on one day, so it was decided by her support team that she could handle it every day. Another one was the school assembly, by some miracle Thea handled a whole school assembly once, even though she has extreme noise sensitivities and there was no proper seating for her regarding her CP. Again, her support team decided she can handle it every time. We should point out that none of the teachers on Thea's support team had any proper experience in dealing with an Autistic child, least of all a dual-diagnosed Autistic child. By the middle of term 2, we removed Thea from the school for her own safety and mental health. We tried contacting the principal, who protected her staff and didn't want to listen to the issues at hand. We then contacted the metro regional office, who just passed the details on to the principal and we received the same response again. Things changed when we contacted Autism Hub, the Department of Education's new unit that was set up to assist schools in educating children on the Spectrum. We actually got a result and spoke to the new coach, who was a familiar face for us – she was the former guidance officer that helped us get Oisin into his special school.

We filled her in on everything and she made an appointment to visit the school on our behalf. During this time, Thea was still away from the school. A couple of weeks passed, and the meeting went ahead. It lasted over three hours, and a lot of positive outcomes came about. The meeting was held on a Friday, and on the following Tuesday the principal reached out to us and asked to meet. We met with her and the Head of Inclusion and a lot was discussed, with positive steps going forward and an apology. Thea returned to school the following day, and we started seeing a change for the rest of term 2.

Unfortunately, there was yet more changes, and not for the better. The Head of Inclusion announced to us that she was moving schools after she had been offered a permanent full-time role at another school and would be leaving at the end of the term. Thea was also losing her mainstream teachers as they were both going on maternity leave (within a week of each other). At the beginning of term 3, Thea had her 3rd Inclusion Officer of the year and a new mainstream teacher. All the procedures that had been put in place in term 2 were undone. Thea's new mainstream teacher didn't understand what noise sensory issues were and couldn't understand why Thea was having constant meltdowns due to the noise. Unfortunately, her Inclusion Officer was no better; she seemed to have difficulty understanding what masking is, and when we told her that Thea wasn't coping, she basically told us that she never saw any of the problems that we raised.

So, we pulled Thea out of the school a month early before the end of term 4. We made the call for her own safety, the safety of those around her, and her mental health. Those last weeks, Thea was getting more and more anxious and the slightest thing would trigger an aggressive response.

As we said earlier, we don't disagree with the inclusion policy, we just don't think it should be forced on every student. It should be used as a policy to get children on the spectrum included into schools and not shut in the room in a corner. Children like Thea that struggle with the sensory overload that is a mainstream classroom shouldn't be forced into that environment. We should be helping them and not putting things in place to intensify their sensory overload. We recently contacted the Minister of Education regarding the inclusion policy and how *we* see it. We weren't expecting much, but we received a call from the Department of Education's Disability and Inclusion unit. It was a welcome conversation from the person who actually was involved in the development of the policy. However, a later response from the minister's advisor was less welcoming, as it did not mention our concerns or the failures of the policy. It was just recommended that we continue working with Autism Hub.

Equally, schools need to have constant procedures in place. Thea's school principal has since admitted (again) that a lack of communication is a big problem in the school. She also admitted that she didn't enforce previous agreed plans with new staff as she sees that as micro-managing. She was quite happy to let them do things their own way whether that be good or bad. This is treating our children like guinea pigs and not educating them. Our children deserve more. They deserve a decent education just the same as neurotypical children.

Our previous story saw the positive in what we were going through. We are even more proud of our kids as they have navigated their way through their own trials. If we could change anything it would be to change the world's acceptance of them and how they are engaged and educated. It's not hard or even expensive to provide neurodiverse children with a safe and supportive environment to receive a good education. Unfortunately, the people that make these decisions have no real-world experience and just look at something on a bit of paper and implement it from a desk (and we were told this by the Department of Education).

We have one more year left for Thea, and then she's off to an independent high school where we hope things will better for her. It's a school that specialises in educating children that struggle with the mainstream environment. Oisin is starting middle school next year, and although he's anxious we're hopeful that he'll transition okay. Oscar is going into Year 1. This'll be the last year that he's in the same school as his sister, and we know it'll be bittersweet for them both.

We are just at another milestone in our journey, but not the end ...

PAUL AND RACHAEL RENDLE *are married and living in Brisbane, Australia. They have been together for 15 years and have three children. Two of their children have special needs: their 11-year-old daughter has a Cerebral Palsy diagnosis as well as being Autistic, and their nine-year-old son is also Autistic and has an intellectual impairment.*

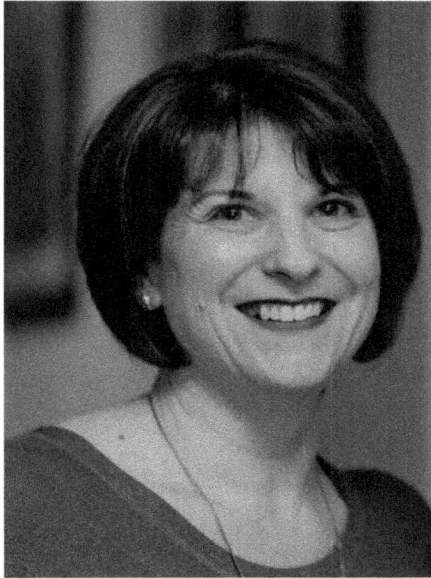

Growing and Learning, but Still So Very Proud
by E. Sal

It's now been a few years since I wrote *Small Things, Big Pride* in the first book of *Parenting A Child on the Spectrum*, and at that time we were just a few short years into knowing that we were living with ASD in our home. We were only starting to understand and recognise the ways in which our Little Miss's brain was wired and what her different (and often unpredictable) responses and reactions really meant.

Mostly, if I'm totally honest, I was tired. Like completely mentally and physically drained, tired. I was overwhelmed by the prospect of a lifetime of this journey and how I was going to 'keep it all together' and 'get us through'. Then, while I was writing our story for the book *Parenting A Child on the Spectrum*, we experienced the first big turning point. I can now look back and say it really was the first of many, but the day of what we have come to call the 'great lunchbox breakthrough' stills sticks in my mind as the moment my energy levels started to lift and I began to see a future that would be less overwhelming and heart-breaking.

Just a few months ago, my gorgeous Miss ASD asked to read 'the story in the book you wrote about me'. I pulled the book down from the shelf, found the page and passed it to Tahlia with some trepidation as to what her response might be. I watched intently as her eyes darted across the lines of text, held my tongue as she turned the pages and then braced myself as her eyes began to glisten followed by a stream of flowing tears.

I was gutted!

I shouldn't have let her read it.

It's upset her too much.

How am I supposed to fix this now?

When she finished reading and closed the book, taking a very deep breath, I asked her if reading the story had upset her too much. She shook her head, but the tears were still flowing, and she was hugging herself tightly. It was another one of those moments when I felt a little lost as her parent, uncertain of how to help her.

I gave her a moment and then asked, as gently as I could, what had upset her so much? 'I'm not upset Mummy,' came the quiet reply. I asked then why she was crying and my heart simultaneously broke and overflowed as she said, 'It's just that you love me so much!'

When I first began thinking about writing this follow up to our story, I checked in with Tahlia that she would be alright with it. She enthusiastically gave me nods of delight and encouraged me to put pen to paper. Next, I deliberated on all that has happened in our lives since the great lunchbox breakthrough and the journey we are all still on.

Tahlia is about to enter her final year of primary school at a fantastic mainstream school which we are very grateful to live within walking distance of. Both our girls have spent their entire early school years at the one education haven which has been fantastic for our whole family.

In all the ways that these things are measured, Tahlia is so successfully competent and accomplished. She is academically ahead, community minded, kind and generous, plays in the school band, reaches amazing heights in her chosen team sport (literally – she is a cheerleading fly), and, in all areas, has received numerous accolades and awards. To our delight, her teachers rate her very highly in the area of social skills and communication, and we know her to be (mostly) socially aware and active.

I feel the need to detour here slightly. Nothing upsets me more than the expectations of our society that ASD means a person can't, or won't be able to, achieve in certain areas. When extended family comment on Tahlia's successes or achievements through the obvious undercurrent of 'even though she has ASD', all my hairs simultaneously prickle. So, please, don't mistake my comments at the end of the previous paragraph. I don't write about her social skills and friendships because I am surprised by it or wasn't expecting it, but rather my delight is a result of growing up myself as the most teased (and bullied) child of the school playground (and classroom) until I changed schools when I was the same age Tahlia is now.

So, in every way seen by the outside world, Tahlia is doing great! At home though, in her 'safe place', with those that love and understand her the most, Tahlia's difficulties all come rushing to the fore. Here she 'lets it all go' and struggles with communication, task management, executive functioning and social etiquette. We find ourselves in a constant round of changing strategies and supports in an effort to help us each manage and cope on the home front.

I find though that it's most difficult for her older sister, Madeline, as she tries to help and make things easier for everyone. With less than 2 years of extra life experience, Madeline becomes increasingly frustrated and alternately jealous of the support and attention her younger sister needs. Add to that Madeline's own transitioning to high school, entering the teenage years of angst and hormones, and our house can often resemble a bomb site – both physically and emotionally. I find myself needing to take a time out in my bedroom more and more often over the last few months!

This season of our family life, tough as it may be, has brought its own set of benefits and understandings too, though. I've come to better understand the part that stress plays on Tahlia's abilities and difficulties. In turn, I've also come to witness how, in dealing with the stress, her need to find and have control creates stress for those of us that love her most – especially her sister.

If I'm honest, that would be the biggest lesson I have gotten from having ASD in our home. I am by nature an organised person that loves to plan and strategise. While this has served our family well in terms of managing the day-to-day running of a house and two young growing children, it also lends me towards frustration and stress when the plans and strategies don't quite work out; and when ASD is involved, let's be honest, things can regularly turn to mayhem and chaos, despite the best preparations.

Over the last couple of years in particular, I have found myself having to consciously change my mindset and work on my resulting behaviours and way of being so that our family can find our way back 'onto the rails' faster and with as little residual angst as possible. In my quiet times, I often reflect on how different (and better, I hope) a Mum I have become due to the teachings and lessons I have gotten from Tahlia and her ASD brain. This has been great for everyone, and I am forever grateful for ASD's presence in our home for my newfound (and growing) ability to remain calmer through the chaos. I am intensely aware that this enables me to be a much better role model for both my girls.

Lately, observing how the two of them interact, especially when they aren't aware that I am watching, has helped me to realise that a lot of their relationship issues are most likely just normal sibling rivalry at its worst. Without a 'control' for this 'experiment' of how child-raising works in our family, how fair is it to blame ASD and its presence in our lives for all the stresses and struggles we face?

And does it even matter what the cause behind why our parenting and family journey looks like this is? Surely what is most important is the lessons and growth we each take on, and support each other through, as individuals with our own difficulties and strengths, both expected and surprising.

In amongst all the literature Josh and I first poured over way back when Tahlia was first diagnosed with ASD, there was a story I find myself constantly coming back to. It talks of booking a most-wanted holiday to a favourite location. Spending months preparing and getting excited, only to find yourself stepping off the plane in a completely different place. It may not be the holiday you had planned for, but it can still be a great holiday. ASD can be just like that; it's not necessarily the parenting journey you had imagined for you and your child, but that doesn't mean it has to be any less wonderful. I enjoy the most rewarding relationships with both my girls, filled with love and pride.

I was discussing the holiday story and my subsequent realisation with a friend recently, and she made the very valid point that parenting is like that with every child – ASD or not. They all have different personalities and difficulties and phases that result in the reality of your journey together never fitting the mould of what you imagined it would be.

And there are some great lessons for us as parents, and for our personal growth, if we can learn to be present to the life and relationships we have, instead of being disappointed that it doesn't look or feel like what our imagination dreamed up years ago. Raising a child with ASD has encouraged me – no, let's be real, *forced* me – to control my impulse to 'lose it', scream and heighten the brewing storm. I have had to become a calmer, more controlled person – and I am so much happier this way.

This has permeated into every area of my life and as a result my relationships are much stronger, and I have so much more energy and zest for life. In turn, I am now able to 'see' things I was blind to before, like the circle of stress in our home and the impact it has on each individual, as well as each of our parts in creating and/or abating the brewing storms. This next stage in my gained understanding of how to be the best parent I can is stretching me to grow again as I support each member of my family through this phase of emotional turmoil.

So that brings me back to the question of *Parenting A Child on the Spectrum* and what insights I might have for those just starting out on this journey. For all that I have said about the parenting of every child being different to that which we as parents have imagined, there are certain common experiences that parents of children with ASD seem to all relate to. And it is hard. And it is tiring. And it most definitely is energy draining and mentally fatiguing. But we are not alone. We are not the only one in the whole world with a child that struggles or has difficulties. You are not the only one that has faced the road ahead of you and those of us further ahead are here to help and support you.

My biggest piece of advice would have to be: Look – After – You. One of our specialists once told me I need to be 'selfish'. At the time I internally revolted at the idea – that is not how I wanted to parent, putting my needs above theirs. I now understand the *necessity* in putting myself first and foremost. My health, my mindset, my wellbeing, my energy levels, my ability to be the best version of me to be able to cope with the life of raising two girls, one who happens to be on the spectrum.

Before finishing writing this next step in our story, I took a moment to re-read my original story again. I think the best way to finish this update is to let you all know that we have all come a long way, and yet I am aware that we are only still at the start of our journey. I can honestly reflect over where we have come from, where we have been, and where we are now, and still say, as I did a few years ago, that I am so very proud of us!

E. SAL lives in Melbourne with her husband, their two beautiful girls and their pet lizard. She works part-time and also runs a successful business guiding people from all walks of life from around the globe in the areas of Mindful Matters and Intentional Parenting. She writes to help maintain her sanity.

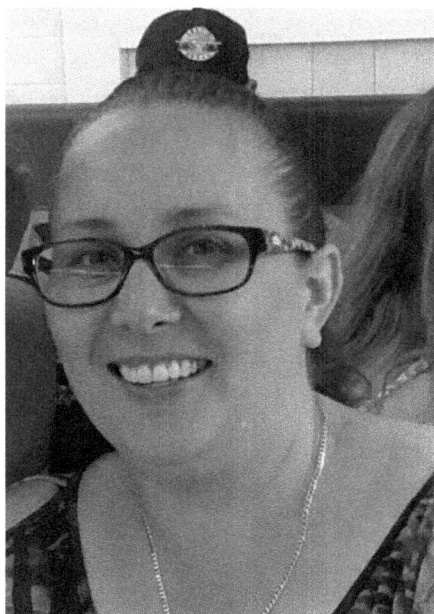

Walking Together, Learning Together
by Alison Carney

When I first shared our story, we were at the stage where we had just started working on strategies and learning about what ASD was and how this would look for our family, as we all know being on the spectrum looks different for everyone. To recap, Jacob was in his second year of high school, Caleb was heading towards his senior year in primary school and Dylan was in his first year of school. We were still finding our feet and discovering that routine and communication were key.

Fast forward four years, and all of a sudden you realise just how much can be achieved in such a short amount of time. We spent lots of money on different appointments and receiving support and advice from many different sources, we did have to decide which ones were beneficial and which ones would go as it gets very expensive. We preferred the paediatrician and the psychologist and found this worked for the boys. Sadly, as Caleb grew older and was able to understand more, we had to stop the psychologist for him and focus on getting Dylan to where he needed to be. This did affect Caleb a little, but he is very understanding, and we worked with him using a lot of the strategies that were already in place. Some of these strategies included visual lists around the house to help remind him of certain things without having to overwhelm him by nagging, and also allowing him to help plan the routines so he was part of the process and felt he was in control of his own actions.

The appointments eventually stopped for Dylan also, as my husband and I were now in the process of building a house which was the priority. I don't think the boys suffered too much from this as they were part of the process the whole time. We participated in video interviews and reviews and they were asked questions about the house and what room they would pick. We often stopped by the house and checked on the process. This was a family project and it meant we could settle. We have now been in the house for four years, and since landing on our feet we have been able to get back to focusing on the children and their future.

Jacob has done well with his high school years and is entering his final year now. He has almost completed his 100 hours of driving and will be able to drive on his provisional licence soon. 100 hours has been tough to fit into the schedule, but we made it a priority as this is super important for Jacob to move forward and reach his goals. Jacob is working part-time after school, on weekends and a lot in the school holidays. We have also helped Jacob to learn how to save money so he can buy a car and support himself when needed. Caleb and Dylan really look up to their older brother and he sets a good example; they are also very protective of him and take his side most of the time, so I know their bond is strong. They never hurt each other, and rarely fight. We are so proud of the close bond they all have, and we know no matter what they will always stick together.

Walking Together, Learning Together
by Alison Carney

Caleb often looks forward to following in his brother's footsteps; he always has. His school years have been tough, but we always look for a way to resolve any issues and carry on because that's what we have to do. Caleb started high school at the same school as his brother and it was hard; he would often come home upset and not wanting to go back. After lots of discussion, we discovered that high school for Caleb was a very scary place, the way he saw it and the way he felt while he was there, and it was important that we understood him and looked at it from his point of view. Caleb told us that high school was scary and the people there were kids but they looked and acted like fully grown men, with full faces of hair and loud swearing or talking. These are not the usual reasons that someone is scared to go to school, but for Caleb that was extremely scary, and it was important that we put ourselves in his shoes. We discussed some options with Caleb and asked for his opinion on some of these options. He was involved in making the decision for his future. We also had to remind him that he can't keep changing schools, so whatever decision we came to, we would have to get through it together.

After visiting a few schools and talking about the pros and cons, we settled on a smaller private school. Another cost, but we were willing to accept this as long as Caleb was happy to go to school and do the best he could. Caleb settled in quickly and was accepted by many of his peers, and the support he has received and continues to receive from the school is amazing. Caleb has had some small struggles in high school, but they always work with him to come to a conclusion and they support his struggles and his achievements with no judgement. I honestly feel this has been one of the better decisions we have made with Caleb to get him through his high school years. Caleb is now heading into year 10 and has decided to continue studying psychology. He soaks up all the knowledge from this subject and puts it into practice at home, even with his parents. So not only have we supported Caleb, but he is also supporting us and teaching us so many new skills and helping us to understand our thoughts and emotions. Caleb is also working part time at the same place his brother works. This is an extra challenge, but he does his best and enjoys earning some money while also having a little extra bit of responsibility. Caleb knows what some of his triggers are now, and we often only need to give him a gentle reminder and he will take some time and regroup himself. He is very good to his little brother Dylan as well, and often helps him with his routine while sometimes reminding us to chill.

Dylan has had a tough run with school recently. He started out doing ok in his first couple of years, with the teachers finding or looking for strategies that worked or might work. Dylan struggles a lot in school as he also lives with intellectual impairment, which means that in year 4 he still follows a prep curriculum. As Dylan got older and it became more noticeable to his peers that he was different, and the teachers started to expect more from Dylan, things started to get really tough. I would receive phone calls at work to come and collect him as he had run away and was near the road. One day, I got a call to say he was suspended as he had used a swear word at the principal.

Many of these things were out of character for Dylan, so we arranged to meet with the school and discuss what we could do. We were advised that Dylan did not fit into any of the tiers even after strategies had been put in place, and it was strongly suggested that we medicate Dylan. It was also requested that we pick Dylan up every day at midday, so he did not become too overwhelmed at school. These requests were understandable, but we knew our son was capable of so much more, and we both worked full time, so it was time to reassess and see where to next. We saw the paediatrician and trialled the meds, as we had also done in the past with no success but given that Dylan was older now, we thought we would try again.

One day on meds and Dylan was a wreck; he hid in his tent for the entire day crying about little things and saying, 'I don't know what's wrong'. We did not see even a little bit of hope with this, and knew it was not what was going to work for Dylan. We are aware it may work for many other children, but we know our boy, and this is not what he needed. It was time to look at other options. We know that a smaller private school helped with Caleb, so we tried this for Dylan, but unfortunately the school could not accept Dylan as his needs were too high and they did not want to let him down. We looked into an Autism school, but because of his intellectual impairment they would not accept him. By this stage we were in meltdown mode. Eventually I approached a very small private primary school that was right next to where I work, and after lots of meetings and paperwork, Dylan was accepted at this school and he started in term 3 of year 4.

This was a very scary time for us as we wondered if Dylan would cope with the change, but what reassured us was the effort that the school put in to get to know Dylan before they even accepted him. They visited him at his current school, observing him and trying to ensure they had a clear picture of his needs and how to best support him. They then came to us with their visions and goals for Dylan. We were gobsmacked; they had met our son only a few times, and, through observation and collaboration, we felt like they knew our son the way we knew our son – and right when we were starting to lose hope and doubt ourselves.

Dylan has now been at the school for two terms, and he has a wonderful teacher that treats him equally and encourages and challenges him to achieve the things he knows he can achieve. We feel like we have our little boy back, and the future is looking bright for him. He is learning to read some basic words and he got his first ever award for mathematics. Apparently, he loves to measure everything in the classroom. We are so happy that Dylan is finally able to learn in a way that he understands, and that he is being recognised for his individuality rather than for his disruptiveness. He is making friends and telling us about his day rather than coming home early and being in a state of disrepair.

Through all of this, we have realised the best thing for our children is to listen to their needs and be their advocate, and that what works for one will probably not work for the other. Get to know what each of your children need and support them with this. Yes, it is extra pressure and sometimes a struggle, but our children trust that we will help them get through all of this and help them land on their feet.

We have worked really hard to make sure we try everything we can for the kids, and when we find something that works, we settle and monitor the progress. If something's not working, we try to understand why, and we always talk to the children about it. We are coming into adulthood now with our two oldest and I am sure we will have new struggles, but we are fairly confident that the decisions we have made together are working well for now. I honestly feel that if something isn't working then you need to think about why. The absolute best thing for us recently has been choosing the right schools for all our boys, even though this means 3 different drop offs and not having them at school together. It's ok to have different needs and wants but try not to push those away, embrace them and see where it leads.

*My name is **ALISON CARNEY**, I am a devoted wife and mother to 3 sons. I love to spend time with my immediate family and extended family as they mean the world to me.*

Walking Together, Learning Together
by Alison Carney

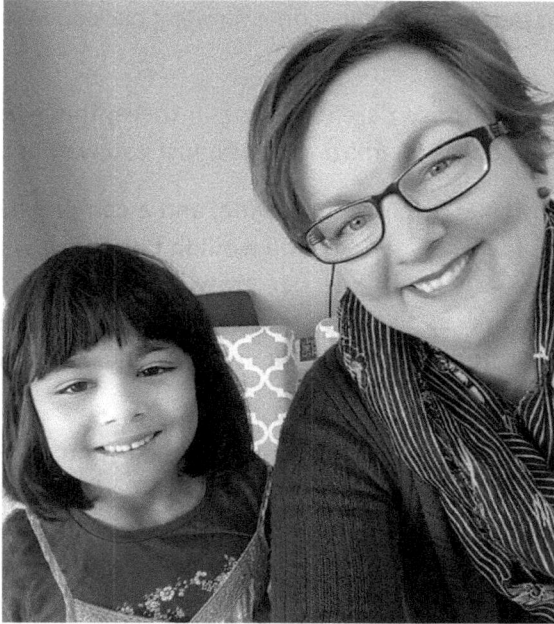

Goodbye to the Warzone
by Fiona Stock

A warzone. That's what I felt I was living in when I wrote my original piece for *Parenting A Child on the Spectrum*. My child was smashing her head against walls. My marriage was awful. I was hanging on by a bare thread. For the most part, I was absorbed in surviving the moment. If ever I dared to look ahead, I couldn't tell if it would get better, or if this was just it.

Miserable. Awful.

When I see mums now struggling through those days, when I recognise the overwhelm that lies behind their outwardly coping exterior, it brings tears to my eyes. Sometimes, when I see a child having a dreadful meltdown, those feelings of helplessness and despair come flooding back and I want to burst into tears.

But I also want to tell those parents: 'Hang in there, this will pass. It will get better. And your child will do amazing things. Just you wait and see.'

Because today, my child is happy, achieving, and a completely different being to that screaming, raging 3-year-old. You wouldn't believe it was the same child if you hadn't been around to see her grow. She is smart, communicative, outgoing, joyful... quirky as all get-up, and unable to ever be still... but our lives are peaceful more often than not. Here are just some of the things that have changed for the better:

- My daughter no longer has a severe communication delay. After years of seemingly intractable receptive language difficulties, we can now hold conversations. Factual ones, not esoteric, but I still feel the miracle of this.
- My daughter can now cope with changes to plans, will try new and challenging things and is amazingly resilient. She has coped with her parents' divorce and sharing time between two houses better than I ever would have expected.
- My daughter no longer presents as having an intellectual disability and is transitioning from special school to mainstream school. It turns out she actually has a great brain for maths, science, reading and remembering a multitude of facts.
- For all the NDIS system's flaws, the funding has allowed us to participate in extra-curricular activities and given me some much-needed respite.

Most important of all, my beautiful girl is happy. She is no longer a ball of raging, anxiety-ridden frustration. We understand each other well now and have built a life that revolves around meeting her needs. One up-side of no longer being married is I only have one other person's complex needs to attend to, and full-blown meltdowns are few and far between. While life is not exactly easy – I am a single mum living on the breadline and juggling 99% of the child-related stuff, after all – for the most part our life is good. When I'm not completely exhausted, I take real pleasure in my funny, beautiful, bright little girl's left-of-centre antics.

Something wonderful has also been happening in the Autism world since I last wrote. It is the growing neurodiversity movement, coupled with the increasingly heard voice of autistics*. What if, the neurodiversity movement posits, Autism wasn't a mistake or a tragedy, but rather a different neurology in a whole world of varying neurologies? What if the autistic mind isn't 'wrong', it's actually a treasure that enriches the world? I like this view. I like the notion that my daughter is 'Different, Not Less', as they say. I now see her strengths, and how valuable they can be. For example, my daughter has an incredible memory for names, places, dates... all things I am hideously bad at remembering. How useful to have a daughter that can remind me of people's names! She will also spot the thing that's out of place, which is a very useful skill, for example, in workplaces that need to spot errors in screen upon screen of coding.

The internet has been the perfect vehicle for people who are socially awkward or struggle to communicate verbally, or quickly, to get their thoughts out into the world. It has also allowed autistics to find each other, and to discuss things without the interference of dominant neurotypical perspectives. Eavesdropping on adult autistics is incredibly helpful to parents like me, when we struggle to understand what's happening inside our child's head. They can explain for us what sensory overload feels like, they can help us understand how our little person might view a situation. And I can tell you, more than any therapy we have undertaken, my increased ability to understand my daughter's perspective has helped us most of all.

There is a flip-side – for eons, us neurotypicals have had things all our way. Now the autistic side is fighting back and claiming their space. This is a good and necessary thing, but our community is also riven with schisms. Neurotypicals vs autistics, ABA therapy proponents vs those that believe it's tantamount to torture. Those that insist on person-first use of 'person with Autism' vs those that advocate 'autistic person' or 'autistics'. As with every other discourse on the internet, battles feel pitched and punches are not always pulled.

The thing I personally find hard is the question of whether a parent should publicly talk about how difficult raising their child with Autism is. From the autistic perspective, doing so continues to feed the predominant narrative that Autism is 'awful' and 'wrong'. Hearing that message over and over again as they grow up, autistic people have much higher rates of mental health issues and even suicide. But on the flip side, from the parent's perspective, to pretend that everything is OK is to lie about the depth of difficulty of raising an autistic child. When we are crying out for support, to remain silent runs the risk of muting our message. And dammit, sometimes we just need people to acknowledge our experience and sympathise! It is a hard thing to be told we are betraying our children by airing our grievances, when we feel that we are giving so much of ourselves to champion them.

But still, I listen to autistic voices, and I try to honour them. Because it is important that the narrative changes and our children are recognised as the valuable people that they are. And as parents, our role needs to be one of boundless support, encouragement, and belief in our children's potential.

It's Not All Flowers and Sunshine

That's the positive bit, and what I wanted this whole chapter to be like.

But now, as I continue writing, something awful happens. A rant pours out.

I have tried writing about school, and before I know it, 1000 words of rant have spewed onto the page.

I have started talking about extra-curricular activities, and more vitriolic language about a lack of inclusion has poured from my pen.

Goodbye to the Warzone
by Fiona Stock

I didn't realise I was so pissed off about things! While you could say I'm far more positive about Autism these days, I've become much more jaded about our society in general.

In my day-to-day life, I am the epitome of calm. When the teacher calls me aside at pick-up time to tell me what transgression has transpired that day, I listen impassively. When yet another dance or sports class doesn't work out, I take it on the chin. When my daughter loses the plot and can't be consoled, I wait it out without expressing my own frustration.

But it seems that, underneath it all, I actually have raging anger issues.

Because to be perfectly honest, being that calm person when challenge after challenge is hurled at you is exhausting and frustrating and highly annoying.

It's the challenges of finding a place in our society that drive me most to distraction. Trying to fit an autistic child into a school system that doesn't support them – something the government knows but does little to change. Trying to participate in after-school activities where management are so terrified of what might be required to support inclusion that they'd rather just say 'no' than meet me to discuss the possibilities. Trying to keep a roof above our heads when I'm too busy attending to my child's needs/schooling issues/dealing with NDIS requirements to work full time, but don't qualify for a carer's pension and no longer have enough fight left in me to force the issue any further with Centrelink.

I could write about all these circumstances at length, but I'd need a whole book and it would probably be a very boring one. Suffice to say, I always used to think Australia had a great social support system for people in need, and that our education system catered pretty well for all. I now know different, and it is a huge shock to me to find out how incredibly incompetent and perverse our Centrelink, schooling, child support and disability support systems can be. I give thanks that I am not raising a child with Autism in an actual warzone or as a refugee, but still I know things can and should be better.

The Problem with Schooling

Not every parent wants their child with additional needs to be included in a mainstream school. When my daughter was turning 5, I just knew it wouldn't be the right place for her, whereas the local special school offered the kind of support she needed.

However, you can't just choose the type of school your child goes to. It all depends on an IQ test administered by the Department of Education – score under 70 and you are eligible for special school. Over that, and you're off to mainstream. There are also Autism specific schools available, but their entry requirement is significantly delayed communication. And even if you meet their criteria, insufficient places mean you still may miss out on a spot.

This system is terrible for many autistic kids who may not have a low enough IQ to be eligible for the special school system, may not have the communication delays required for the Autism specific school, and who also don't qualify for funded support in the mainstream system (who are often reluctant to take them). Where, then, do they fit?

To make things worse, those all-important IQ tests don't actually work well for kids on the spectrum. My daughter is a case in point. At age 5, she simply couldn't engage with the tester enough to produce any kind of result, and I had to argue that yes, she was intelligent enough to attend special school, and not the next tier down. Two years later, when she was tested again, and despite running out of the room and twirling all over the place during the test, she scored too high to remain in special school, and was effectively booted into the mainstream system. Same kid. Presumably, the same IQ. Two vastly different results.

The irony, of course, is she tested so much better the second time around, precisely because she was in a schooling environment that had enabled her to thrive. But now that fabulous progress meant tackling a schooling system that I knew wouldn't cater for her needs.

I was gutted, and terrified. And, after ringing all the local schools and hearing all the excuses why they could not accept my child or support her if she did enrol (an attitude that is totally illegal but disgustingly common), I despaired.

When I finally heard the words, 'your daughter will be welcome here and, even if she doesn't come with any funding, we will do whatever we can to support her' from a mainstream school principal, I remained seemingly unmoved while I exited the office, then cried in relief once I reached the car.

Meanwhile, the principal of her special school helped me appeal to the Department of Education for another two years of transition time, and we started on the journey of dual enrolment. My daughter now attends both special and mainstream schools each week and will transition to mainstream school full time by the end of this year.

It has been scary, fraught with weekly difficulties, and I'm still not entirely convinced my daughter is best off in mainstream school, but she has surprised me with her continued progress and delight in her new school. My worst fears have not come to pass.

But it is an ongoing battle. There are days when my daughter loses the plot and hits her aide or refuses to set foot in her mainstream classroom. And while the teachers try hard, they simply do not have the specialist knowledge nor the teacher-to-student ratios that the special schools have. My child does not often follow along with the rest of the class, does not get included in the playground like a regular kid, and I routinely have to spend time discussing issues with her teachers. To be honest, sometimes I long to just pick up my kid like every other parent and not have to hear about issues that occurred that day.

The miracle of it all is she is such a clever child, in her own way, that she still learns at an amazing pace. She memorised an entire song in Chinese in one lesson. Just for fun, she asks me to give her complicated maths sums involving negative numbers or algebra for her to do in her head. She has been able to read pretty much every word of the English language for several years now.

The flipside of this, though, is current educational methods don't support her learning style. Maths problems are written out in words instead of equations, which makes it hard for her to do them, and subsequently she gets set overly simple goals like 'she will be able to recognise a 3-digit number'. She refuses to read the set texts, or can't answer comprehension questions, so gets set babyish readers. But my girl doesn't learn in a linear pattern from simple to complex. No, she learns by memorising the complex, at first not understanding, but one day a lightbulb goes off and she suddenly gets it. Deny her access to that higher level by insisting she work her way up there, and she's going to languish at the bottom. I sometimes feel like school is something she just has to get through before she can find her real place in the world.

All this is to say... our schooling system is *not* set up to support our autistic kids. Everyone knows it, the government has been looking into it, but so far nothing has changed. I do believe it will. But for now, huge swathes of autistic children fall behind, drop out, parents are forced to home-school, society suffers for it, and we all lose a whole lot of potential.

But There Are Angels

For all that the systems are unwieldy, we have found golden individuals along the way, and they make all the difference in the world. A wonderful speech pathologist, who was always thinking how to make exercises more exciting. A kinder teacher willing to change the way she did things despite decades of experience. The most amazing special school; a principal who says, 'Yes, you are welcome here.' The local Girl Guides troop, whose aim of inclusion for every girl has meant we have found a place to fit in.

While the big systems fail our kids, individuals catch their fall and lift them up. And more and more, they have fellow autistics alongside to help. Autistic-led mentoring and social groups, such as the I Can Network and Yellow Ladybugs, are providing spaces for autistic kids to belong, and encouragement for us parents as we see what capable people our children can grow up to be. When I look forward, I can see societal attitudes changing, employment opportunities opening up, and I actually feel pretty positive about my little girl's future. I feel like my child has so much potential inside her, just waiting to explode out and be seen. I hope that she comes into her own as a young adult and can tread her own path and find meaningful employment that plays on her strengths. And of course, I pray that one day she will find friends and a partner who understand and love her in all her quirky glory.

*Note: I have chosen to use the phrase 'autistic person' rather than 'person with Autism'. Many parents and educators use 'person with Autism', to reflect the fact that they see the person first, not their diagnosis. However, many autistic people now prefer 'autistic person' because Autism is intrinsic to their identity. There is no current consensus on which term is correct, so I have chosen to go with the term most commonly used by the people I believe we should listen to most – those who are actually autistic.

FIONA STOCK is a Melbourne-based mum of one gorgeous, zany, active 8-year-old girl with Autism who currently has no front teeth and enjoys gymnastics, girl guides, science experiments and making endless artistic creations out of folded paper. Fiona wrote in the original Parenting A Child on the Spectrum *under her married name Fiona Amarasinghe but has since divorced and now lives in a cosy little apartment with her daughter (who also spends time at dad's place). Fiona has a wildly varied work history, ranging from management consulting to belly dancing to running her own children's party business. She now cobbles together a sort-of living working as a writer-for-hire for small businesses and doing administrative tasks – basically anything that can be done within school hours and provide the flexibility needed to keep her daughter happy and well.*

www.ingramcontent.com/pod-product-compliance
Lightning Source LLC
Chambersburg PA
CBHW072136020426
42334CB00018B/1831